Anaphylaxis
A Practical Guide

Philip Jevon RN BSc(Hons) PGCE
Resuscitation Training Officer, Manor Hospital, Walsall, UK

With Chapter II written by
Bridgit Dimond MA LLB DSA AHSM Barrister-at-law
Emeritus Professor, University of Glamorgan, UK

Consultant Editors
Jonathan North MB BCh FRCPath DM
Consultant Immunologist, City Hospital, Birmingham, UK

David F Bowden FRCS FFAEM
Consultant in Accident and Emergency Medicine
Manor Hospital, Walsall, UK

Jagtar Singh Pooni BSc(Hons) FRCP(UK) FRCA
Consultant in Anaesthetics and Intensive Care, New Cross Hospital,
Wolverhampton, UK

Foreword by
Richard S H Pumphrey FRCPath
Immunology Consultant, St. Mary's Hospital,
Manchester, UK

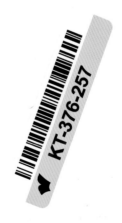

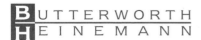
BUTTERWORTH
HEINEMANN

EDINBURGH LONDON NEW YORK OXFORD PHILADELPHIA ST LOUIS SYDNEY TORONTO 2004

BUTTERWORTH-HEINEMANN
An imprint of Elsevier Limited

First published 2004

ISBN 0 7506 8788 6

British Library Cataloguing in Publication Data
A catalogue record for this book is available from the British Library

Library of Congress Cataloging in Publication Data
A catalog record for this book is available from the Library of Congress

Notice
Knowledge and best practice in this field are constantly changing. As new
research and experience broaden our knowledge, changes in practices,
treatment and drug therapy may become necessary or appropriate. Readers
are advised to check the most current information provided (i) on
procedures featured or (ii) by the manufacturer of each product to be
administered, to verify the recommended dose or formula, the method
and duration of administration, and contraindications. It is the responsibility
of the practitioner, relying on their own experience and knowledge of the
patient, to make diagnoses, to determine dosages and the best treatment
for each individual patient, and to take all appropriate safety precautions.
To the fullest extent of the law, neither the Publisher nor the author
assumes any liability for any injury and/or damage.

The Publisher

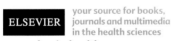

your source for books,
journals and multimedia
in the health sciences
www.elsevierhealth.com

The
Publisher's
policy is to use
**paper manufactured
from sustainable forests**

Printed in China

Contents

Foreword

Allergy is now so common that more than a third of those living in the UK have it to a lesser or greater extent. Each year 20–30 people out of our population of 60 million die from acute reactions – and most of these did not even know they had an allergy until the fatal reaction. This book is about how to recognise and treat those who have the most severe acute reactions – anaphylaxis.

Scientists have to take care that the words they use have exact meanings that are understood in the same way by everyone in the field. Unfortunately, 'anaphylaxis' is one of those terms whose meaning has changed alongside the understanding of immune responses over the years. It was coined by Charles Richet in 1902 to denote the unexpected increase in sensitivity of experimental animals to coelenterate toxins following exposure to a sublethal dose; he intended the term to convey the converse of prophylaxis. It soon became clear that it was not an increase in toxicity but rather a self-destructive immune reaction – a form of hypersensitivity as it was later to become known.

Once the type of antibody involved in anaphylaxis was understood, it became possible to investigate the allergy underlying these reactions by measuring the IgE antibody level against the allergen triggering the reactions. This spawned a new set of problems: IgE antibodies were not present for all reaction trigger factors, leading to the concept of non-IgE-mediated anaphylaxis, or anaphylactoid reactions as they were called. IgE antibodies caused reactions by stimulating histamine-containing cells to release their histamine and secrete a variety of other potent mediators. Some of these anaphylactoid reactions were caused by agents that triggered the release of mast cell mediators without IgE antibodies, and other anaphylactoid reactions were caused by different pathways that resulted in rapid reactions with some similar features to anaphylaxis, without involving mast cells or basophils.

In 2001 the Nomenclature Committee of the European Association for Allergy and Clinical Immunology (EAACI) published a revised nomenclature for many allergy terms. The Committee wished to use the term anaphylaxis both for the state of altered immunity in which an anaphylactic reaction might occur, as well as a name for the reaction. They defined anaphylaxis as '*a severe, life-threatening, generalised or systemic hypersensitivity reaction*' (EAACI, 2001)

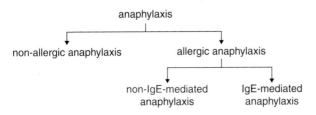

Anaphylaxis was divided first into allergic and non-allergic, and allergic anaphylaxis into IgE-mediated and non-IgE-mediated (Figure). Unfortunately this revised nomenclature has not found favour in the USA, where 'anaphylactoid' is regarded too useful a term to jettison.

Anaphylaxis is unexpectedly difficult to diagnose: it may not be possible to classify a reaction within these definitions, or even know if what happened was anaphylaxis.

There is a continuous spectrum of severity of allergic reactions: inclusion criteria have varied between studies. There is no entirely satisfactory index of severity for anaphylactic reactions. The commonly used grades (Ring & Messmer, 1977) are based on a preconception of which symptoms are likely to occur in reactions of four grades of severity; this does not reflect the continuous spectrum seen in practice. Nor does it take into account the different patterns of symptoms caused by different triggers for reactions. For example, reactions to stings may be fatal because of shock or upper airway swelling, whereas fatal reactions to foods have largely been asthmatic. Mild allergic reactions may include a variety of symptoms including wheezing, rhinitis, conjunctivitis, vomiting, diarrhoea, urticaria, angioedema, difficulty swallowing due to swelling in the throat and so on. The most severe reactions have often only had one or two of these, the whole progressing so rapidly that many features have no time to develop. Often too, anaphylaxis is accompanied by panic. All of this makes it unexpectedly difficult to recognise in time to give optimal treatment.

This little book takes a practical approach to recognising and treating anaphylactic reactions. I hope that reading it will help you to save lives.

References

EAACI (2001) EAACI revised nomenclature for allergy. Allergy 56(9): 813–24

Ring J, Messmer K (1977) Incidence and severity of anaphylactoid reactions to colloid volume substitutes. Lancet 8009: 466–69

Dr Richard Pumphrey
Manchester 2004

Basic physiology of allergy

Introduction

Anaphylaxis is a severe allergic or hypersensitivity reaction, the extreme end of the spectrum of clinical allergy. To understand the mechanisms of anaphylaxis and to appreciate the treatment strategies, it is important to understand the physiology of allergy.

The aim of this chapter is to understand the basic physiology of allergy. If a more detailed account is required Roitt's *Essential Immunology* (1997) is recommended.

Chapter objectives

At the end of the chapter the reader will be able to:

- Define allergy
- Discuss the classification of hypersensitivity reactions
- List the key components of an IgE-mediated hypersensitivity reaction
- Describe the mechanism of an IgE-mediated hypersensitivity reaction
- List the signs and symptoms of an IgE-mediated hypersensitivity reaction
- State the benefits of an IgE-mediated hypersensitivity reaction.

Definition of allergy

'The term allergy is used to describe a response, within the body, to a substance, which is not necessarily harmful in itself, but results in an immune response and a reaction that causes symptoms and disease in a predisposed person' (Allergy UK, 2003a). Basically, allergy is an exaggerated response by the immune system to an external substance (Kay, 2000).

In the UK, approximately 1 in 6 of the population is affected by an allergy or allergies (Kay, 2000) and the incidence is rising (Davies, 1999 and Jarvis & Burney, 2000). The commonest type of allergy involves atopy (Holgate, 2001).

Atopy is derived from the Greek word *atopos*, meaning 'out of place'. It is defined as the production of specific immunoglobulin E (IgE) antibodies which, by having a strong affinity for mast cells and basophils, provide a mechanism for hypersensitivity reactions through the release of proallergic chemicals from these cells (Holgate, 2001). This reaction may be mild, producing symptoms such as sneezing or a runny nose, or severe, resulting in life-threatening anaphylaxis (Jones, 2002).

Atopy is not an illness but an inherited feature, which makes individuals more susceptible to the development of an allergic disorder (Allergy UK, 2003a). Atopy is closely linked to allergic diseases such as asthma, hayfever and eczema. However, not everyone with atopy develops clinical manifestations of allergy, and not everyone with clinical features compatible with allergy is shown to be atopic when tested for specific IgE antibodies to a broad range of environmental allergens (Jarvis & Burney, 2000).

A person who is overly reactive to a drug or a substance that is tolerated by most other people is said to be hypersensitive.

Classification of hypersensitivity reactions

Hypersensitivity reactions are classified into four types (1, 2, 3 and 4), depending on their mechanisms:

- **Type I hypersensitivity reaction:** triggering of mast cells by IgE. Sometimes referred to as anaphylactic hypersensitivity (Roitt, 1997).
- **Type II cytotoxic hypersensitivity reaction:** IgM and IgG mediated; involves antibodies directed against allergens on the surface of the body's own cells – this mechanism of cell destruction is similar to the destruction of foreign bacteria or protozoa. An example of this type of hypersensitivity is a reaction to a blood transfusion (Roitt, 1997).
- **Type III immune complex hypersensitivity reaction:** involves allergen–antibody complexes: the allergen is eliminated through phagocytosis by cells of the monocyte–macrophage system (Staines et al., 1993).
- **Type IV delayed-type hypersensitivity reaction:** mediated by T cells alone (no antibody involvement); can take weeks to develop (Staines et al., 1993), though often occurs within 48 hours.

The first three are antibody mediated and tend to be referred to as 'immediate'-type reactions (Roitt, 1997) and the fourth is cell mediated (antibody independent) (Staines et al., 1993) and is often referred to as a 'delayed-type' reaction (Roitt, 1997). In anaphylaxis only type I hypersensitivity reaction is relevant (Henderson, 1998).

Components of an IgE-mediated hypersensitivity reaction

Components of type I hypersensitivity reaction include the causative allergen, mast cells, basophils and IgE antibodies.

Allergen

The term allergen, which is generally preferred to the term antigen (antibody generator), is a substance that can produce a hypersensitive reaction in the body (Hendry & Farley, 2001). Examples of allergens include pollens, animal proteins, food proteins and mites (Leech, 2002). Allergens can gain entry to the body by ingestion, injection, inhalation or absorption through the skin (Henderson, 1998).

The allergen itself is normally harmless. It is usually the immune system itself (and not the allergen) that causes the adverse effects on the body (Waugh & Grant, 2001). The way people respond to allergens varies and is probably genetically determined (Leech, 2002).

A particular allergen will result in the production of IgE antibodies that are specific to that allergen and no other – this is sometimes seen as analogous to 'lock and key' (Hendry & Farley, 2001).

Following the initial exposure to the allergen, the individual becomes sensitised (elicits an IgE response); then, on the second or subsequent exposures the immune system mounts a response which is entirely out of proportion to the perceived threat (an exaggerated version of normal immune function) (Waugh & Grant, 2001). The severity of the reaction can increase with repeated exposure to the allergen (Staines et al., 1993).

Mast cells

Mast cells are located just under the skin, along blood vessels in the connective tissue of all organs (excluding the brain) and in the mucosa of the gastrointestinal and respiratory tracts (Leech, 2002). They are most plentiful in regions that come into contact with the external environment, e.g. the skin, outer surface of the eyes, the linings of the respiratory tract and the digestive tract (Sherwood, 2001).

Although the exact function of mast cells is unknown, they do play an important role in the body's inflammatory response which is vital for recovery (Jones, 2002). The cytoplasm of a resting mast cell is filled with large granules that contain chemical mediators of inflammation, including histamine, heparin and tryptase.

During an IgE-mediated hypersensitivity reaction, mast cells are activated. They then degranulate, causing the release of the chemical mediators in the surrounding tissues, collectively resulting in increased vascular permeability and vasodilation (Zull, 1999). Following degranulation, the mast cells synthesise and produce a new set of granules (Parham, 2000).

Basophils

Basophils (basophilic polymorphonuclear leucocytes) contain similar granules to, and have a similar function to, mast cells (Staines et al., 1993). They act as 'circulating mast cells' and mediate systemic allergic reactions and migrate to the tissues to partake in local allergic reactions (Leech, 2002). As with mast cells, during an IgE-mediated hypersensitivity reaction activated basophils release chemical mediators.

IgE antibodies

Immunoglobulins are proteins that are sometimes referred to as 'antibodies'. There are five different classes of immunoglobulins, each having the prefix 'Ig'.

IgE antibodies are responsible for most allergic responses (Parham, 2000). They are normally found in very small quantities in serum (<0.002% of all immunoglobulins) (Hendry & Farley, 2001).

In allergic patients, levels can increase by as much as 2–10 times (Leech, 2002). Interaction between the allergen and the allergen-specific IgE antibodies on the surfaces of mast cells and basophils triggers a hypersensitivity reaction, which can lead to anaphylaxis.

Mechanism of an IgE-mediated hypersensitivity reaction

Initial sensitisation

After the first exposure to the allergen the body produces allergen-specific IgE antibodies, which adhere to the surfaces of mast cells and basophils (Staines et al., 1993). At this point, the person is said to be sensitised (Hendry & Farley, 2001).

In most cases of anaphylaxis previous exposure to the allergen, together with the formation of allergen-specific IgE antibodies, is a requisite (Zull, 1999) (in the case of anaphylactoid reactions, which are not IgE-mediated, this is not the case (see page 9)).

Hypersensitivity reaction

Following a subsequent exposure, the allergen binds to the allergen-specific IgE antibodies on the surfaces of mast cells and basophils. This cross-linking leads to the degranulation of mast cells and basophils, and hence to the release of chemical mediators, e.g. histamine, tryptase, certain prostaglandins and leukotrienes (Rusznak & Peebles, 2002).

These chemical mediators produce the signs and symptoms of anaphylaxis through their activity on receptors that induce mucus production, pruritus, vascular permeability and smooth muscle constriction in various organs (Rusznak & Peebles, 2002). This release of chemical mediators is usually very rapid (within minutes) (Howarth, 2000).

Late-phase reaction

Sometimes the initial reaction is then followed by a late-phase reaction, which usually begins after 2–4 hours, peaks between 6 and 12 hours and resolves within 24–48 hours (Leech, 2002). This late-phase reaction can be even more profound than the first (Rusznak & Peebles, 2002).

Signs and symptoms of IgE-mediated hypersensitivity reactions

The route of exposure, the allergen, the quantity of allergy, the rate of administration and absorption of the allergen, together with coexisting features such as exercise, can all influence the pattern of an IgE hypersensitivity reaction (Bird, 1996). In addition, the clinical effects of IgE-mediated allergic reactions vary depending on the site of the mast cell activation (Parham, 2000).

Reactions can vary in severity (mild to life-threatening), the onset following allergen exposure can be sudden, but sometimes delayed, and the progress can be slow, rapid or even biphasic (Project Team of The Resuscitation Council (UK), 2002).

For convenience, the signs and symptoms of IgE-mediated hypersensitivity reactions will now be discussed under the four main systems affected. The source for most of the information detailed is Zull (1999).

Respiratory

Rhinitis: symptoms include nasal congestion, generalised irritation of the nose and sneezing; signs include mucosal oedema and rhinorrhea.

Laryngeal oedema: symptoms include hoarseness, dysphagia, 'lump in throat', drooling and asphyxia; signs include inspiratory stridor (high-pitched sound on inspiration) indicative of partial upper airway obstruction, cyanosis, and intercostal and clavicular retractions. Oedema of the lips, tongue, soft palate and uvula may herald concomitant laryngeal oedema.

Bronchospasm: symptoms include cough, chest tightness and dyspnoea (Howarth, 2000); signs include tachypnoea, intercostal and clavicular retractions and wheeze.

Conjunctivitis: symptom is itching; signs include eyelid oedema, tears and conjunctival redness (Leech, 2002).

Cardiovascular

If an allergen enters the circulation, it can cause widespread activation of the mast cells in the connective tissue around the blood vessels. This can lead to an increase in vascular permeability, leakage of plasma, a fall in intravascular volume and peripheral vasodilation, resulting in cardiovascular collapse and shock (Bochner & Lichtenstein, 1991), sometimes referred to as anaphylaxis. Severe hypotension results (Sherwood, 2001). The patient could also develop pallor, tachycardia, and even cardiac arrest (Jevon, 2002).

Examples of how allergens can enter the circulation include:

- Insect sting, e.g. bee or wasp – insect venom
- IV drug administration
- Digested foods containing allergens being rapidly absorbed from the mouth or gut into the circulation
- During surgery – contact with latex gloves worn by the surgeon.

Circulatory shock: symptoms include light-headedness, dizziness, syncope, agitation; signs include tachycardia, pallor, hypotension and oliguria.

Cutaneous

Cutaneous effects can result from direct contact with the allergen, e.g. latex or insect sting, or can arise if the allergen is carried to the skin via the circulation (Parham, 2000).

Urticaria: symptoms include pruritus and flushing; signs include raised wheals on the skin (urticaria literally means 'nettle rash', derived from the Latin word *urtica*, meaning stinging nettles, sometimes referred to as 'hives').

Angioedema: symptoms include non-pruritic tingling and a swollen sensation; signs include non-erythematous, puffy areas of skin that do not pit and which are most prominent on the face and lips (Zull, 1999). Angioedema (swelling of the skin) is caused by increased permeability of subcutaneous blood vessels (Parham, 2000).

Gastrointestinal effects

Degranulation of mast cells in the mucosa of the gastrointestinal tract results in fluid leaving the blood through the now permeable blood vessels, and entering the lumen of the gut (Parham, 2000). Smooth muscle contraction in the gastrointestinal tract results in the expulsion of the allergen, through either vomiting or diarrhoea. In addition, the allergen may be absorbed through the gut wall into the circulation and be transported elsewhere in the body, possibly causing such conditions as urticaria and angioedema (Parham, 2000).

Gastroenteritis: symptoms include colic, abdominal cramps, diarrhoea and vomiting (Zull, 1999).

Benefits of the IgE hypersensitivity reaction

As Staines et al. (1993) comment, 'with all the disadvantages associated with IgE allergic responses, you might ask does IgE actually have a useful function? The answer is that it plays a major role in defence against worms'.

Although the evidence is limited, it is nevertheless widely believed that the IgE-mediated immune response has evolved as a defence against parasites, particularly worms (Parham, 2000 and Sherwood, 2001). Shared characteristics of the immune reactions to allergens and parasite worms include the production of IgE antibodies and an increase in the activity of mast cells and basophils (Sherwood, 2001).

Interestingly, mast cells are mainly concentrated in areas where parasitic worms could enter the body, e.g. the skin, digestive tract and lungs. It has been suggested that the IgE-mediated response is in fact the body's attempt to block the entry of parasites into the body via these routes:

- Inflammatory response in the skin to prevent worms burrowing through it
- Coughing and sneezing to expel worms from the respiratory tract
- Diarrhoea to flush worms out of the digestive system.

Interestingly, epidemiology studies demonstrate that the incidence of allergy in a country increases as parasite incidence decreases (Sherwood, 2001).

Chapter summary

To understand the mechanisms of anaphylaxis and to appreciate the treatment strategies, it is important to understand the basic physiology of allergy. Allergy has been defined and the different hypersensitivity reactions have been classified. The key components of, and the mechanism of, an IgE-mediated hypersensitivity reaction have been described. The signs and symptoms of an IgE-mediated hypersensitivity reaction have been listed.

Chapter 2

Epidemiology

Introduction

The exact prevalence of anaphylaxis in the general population is not known because interpretations of it vary, it is substantially underreported, and only a few epidemiological studies of large populations have been conducted (Rusznak & Peebles, 2002). However, the incidence of anaphylaxis is steadily rising and the most common causes are therapeutic drugs, food and insect stings (Ewan, 2000a).

The aim of this chapter is to help the reader understand the epidemiology of anaphylaxis.

Chapter objectives

At the end of the chapter the reader will be able to:

- Define anaphylaxis
- Outline the historical perspectives of anaphylaxis
- Discuss the incidence of anaphylaxis
- List the causes of anaphylaxis
- Outline the causes of anaphylaxis associated with anaesthesia.

Definition of anaphylaxis

There is no universally accepted definition of anaphylaxis. It comprises a constellation of features, and there is no agreement over what features are essential (Ewan, 2000a). In addition, confusion arises because reactions can be mild, moderate or severe.

A good working definition of anaphylaxis has been proposed by Ewan (2000a): a severe systemic allergic reaction involving respiratory difficulty and/or hypotension, with other clinical features possibly present as well.

The term anaphylactic reaction is commonly used for hypersensitive reactions that are IgE mediated (Project Team of the Resuscitation Council (UK), 2002); i.e. a previous exposure to the allergen has resulted in the formation of IgE antibodies, and on re-exposure a reaction occurs (Jones, 2002).

The term anaphylactoid reaction implies that it is not IgE mediated and not related to prior sensitisation (Howarth & Evans, 1994). Certain substances, e.g. opiates, opaque contrast media and curare, and physical factors such as cold and exercise, can have a direct degranulating effect on mast cells, causing the release of chemical mediators (Zull, 1999).

For simplicity, because both anaphylactic and anaphylactoid reactions present with similar signs and symptoms and the emergency management is identical (Project Team of the Resuscitation Council (UK), 2002), the term anaphylaxis will be used to include both types. The difference is only relevant in the investigatory stage (Ewan, 2000a).

Historical perspectives of anaphylaxis

The first reported case of anaphylaxis could be the sudden death of an Egyptian pharaoh following a bee sting, which was recorded in hieroglyphics in 2640 BC (Bochner & Lichtenstein, 1991).

Sir Thomas Moore recorded that the future King Richard III was aware that strawberries gave him urticaria, and asked for a bowl of the fruit to be served to him at a banquet attended by an arch enemy. When he broke out in a spectacular rash, he accused his guest of trying to poison him and subsequently had him executed (Roitt, 1997).

The term 'anaphylaxis' was first used at the beginning of the last century by Portier and Richet (1902). During an experimental immunisation programme, the researchers observed cases of increased sensitivity instead of the expected protective or prophylactic effect. They referred to this increased sensitivity as anaphylaxis (from the Greek *ana*, meaning backward, and *phylaxis*, meaning protection) (Bochner & Lichtenstein, 1991) – literally meaning 'reverse protection' (Bird, 1996). Quoting Portier and Richet in their own words:

'On board the Prince's yacht, experiments were carried out proving that an aqueous glycerin extract of the filaments of *Physalia* (the jellyfish known as the Portugese Man of War) is extremely toxic to ducks and rabbits. On returning to France I could not obtain *Physalia* and decided to study comparatively the tentacles of *Actinaria* (sea anemone). While endeavouring to determine the toxic dose (of extracts), we soon discovered that some days must lapse before fixing it; for several dogs did not die until the fourth or fifth day after administration or even later. We kept those that had been given insufficient to kill, in order to carry out a second investigation upon these when they had recovered. At this point an unforeseen event occurred. The dogs, which had recovered, were intensely sensitive and died a few minutes after the administration of small doses.

The most typical experiment, that in which the result was indisputable, was carried out on a particularly healthy dog. It was given at first 0.1 ml of the glycerin extract without becoming ill. 22 days later, as it was in perfect health, I gave it a second injection of the same amount. In a few seconds it was extremely ill; breathing became distressful and panting; it could scarcely drag itself along, lay on its side, was seized with diarrhoea, vomited blood and died in 25 minutes.' (Roitt, 1997).

Another early description of the mechanism of an allergic reaction was provided in 1921 by Prausnitz and Kustner, who demonstrated that a serum factor from an allergic person could sensitise normal skin. The serum from a person allergic to fish was injected into the skin of a person who was not: a skin test with fish at this injection site resulted in an immediate wheal and flare response (Staines et al., 1993).

At about the same time, the causes of anaphylactic reactions came under close scrutiny. This period saw the development of a number of heterologous antisera against bacterial toxins, e.g. diphtheria and tetanus, and these became recognised as the most common causes of anaphylaxis in humans (Lamson, 1924).

Incidence of anaphylaxis

The incidence of anaphylaxis is increasing (Sheikh & Alves, 2000, Wilson, 2000 and Gupta et al., 2003), probably linked to an appreciable rise in the prevalence of allergic disease over the last 20–30 years (Project Team of the Resuscitation Council (UK), 2002).

Unfortunately, there are no reliable epidemiological data available concerning anaphylaxis, probably owing to the lack of a universal definition (Project Team of the Resuscitation Council (UK), 2002). Data that are available are often quite variable (Ewan, 2000a). Highlights from recent reports on the incidence of anaphylaxis in the UK include:

- 1:2300 attendees at an Accident & Emergency Department present with anaphylaxis (Stewart & Ewan, 1996).
- Approximately 0.3% of the general population per annum has anaphylaxis (Stewart & Ewan, 1996).
- The incidence of hospital discharge with a primary diagnosis of anaphylaxis increased from 5.6:100 000 in 1991/2 to 10.2:100 000 in 1994/5 (Sheikh & Alves, 2000).
- 1 in 5800 emergency inpatient admissions are attributed to anaphylaxis (Sheikh & Alves, 2001).
- 13 230 admissions for anaphylaxis in England during the period 1990–1 to 2000–1 (Gupta et al., 2003).
- 214 deaths attributed to anaphylaxis in the UK between 1992 and 2001 (Pumphrey, 2004).

A novel approach to study the epidemiology of anaphylaxis was under-taken by Simons et al. (2002a). They examined the injectable adrenaline (epinephrine) dispensing patterns for an out-of-hospital population (1.15 million) in a province in Canada over a 5-year period. They found that, overall, anaphylaxis appeared to peak in early childhood but then gradually declined into old age:

- 0.95% of total population
- 1.44% of <17 years age group
- 0.90% of 17–64 years age group
- 0.32% of >64 years age group
- 5.3% of boys aged 12–17 months (highest dispensing rate).

In infancy, childhood and adolescence, boys were more likely than girls to be dispensed injectable adrenaline (epinephrine): this pattern was reversed in adulthood, although in the elderly dispensing patterns between the sexes were equal.

Anaphylaxis is an important cause of morbidity and mortality (Montanaro & Bardana, 2002). Death from anaphylaxis is becoming more common, particularly in children and young adults (Ewan, 2000a). In the UK, current data suggests that the average annual number of deaths attrib-uted to anaphylaxis is 20.4, most of which are iatrogenic (Pumphrey, 2000).

Causes of anaphylaxis

In adults the leading causes of anaphylaxis are foods, therapeutic drugs, insect venom and latex (Pumphrey & Stanworth, 1996 and Alves & Sheikh, 2001). In children food is the commonest cause (98% in 0–4-year-olds and 94% in 0–18-year-olds), with drugs and insect venom being the cause in a minority of cases (Pumphrey & Stanworth, 1996). The common causes of anaphylaxis will now be discussed.

Food

Foods are a major cause of anaphylaxis (Ewan, 2000a), particularly in the out-of-hospital setting (Shimamoto & Bock, 2003). Most food allergy cases are caused by a relatively small number of foods (Rusznak & Peebles, 2002). Foods commonly associated with anaphylaxis are listed in Box 2.1. Although ingestion is the principal route for food allergens, some highly

---

Box 2.1   Foods commonly associated with anaphylaxis

Peanuts
Tree nuts (e.g. brazil nut)
Fish
Shrimps
Shellfish
Egg
Milk
Sesame

sensitive patients may develop severe symptoms after exposure to minute quantities of allergen by skin contact (Tan et al., 2001).

Nut allergy is the commonest cause of food-related anaphylaxis. The incidence of nut sensitisation has increased by approximately 150% between the late 1980s and the mid-1990s (Tariq et al., 1996 and Grundy et al., 2001). In fact, peanut allergy is the most rapidly increasing acute allergic phenomenon in the UK in the last decade (Hourihane et al., 1996). It is estimated that in the UK 1:200 people have peanut allergy (Moulton & Yates, 1999).

Patients allergic to peanuts are at risk of developing allergy to tree nuts (Ewan, 1996). Patients with anaphylaxis to peas can also have a peanut allergy (Wensing et al., 2003). The main danger with peanut-induced anaphylaxis is the development of laryngeal oedema (Ewan, 1996).

Anaphylactic reactions to food products may occur after exposure to minute quantities of allergen by skin contact (Tan et al., 2001 and Fiocchi et al., 2003). Steensma (2003) described the case of a young woman who was allergic to shrimp and lobster dishes who developed anaphylaxis immediately after kissing her partner, who had just eaten some shrimps.

In children, food accounts for approximately 40% of hospital admissions related to anaphylaxis (Pumphrey & Stanworth, 1996, Novembre et al., 1998 and Alves & Sheikh, 2001). Peanuts and nuts account for 94% of fatal and near-fatal anaphylactic reactions to food (Bock et al., 2001).

Both adults and children can lose their hypersensitivity to a food allergen that causes allergy if the food is correctly identified and eliminated from the diet for 1–2 years (Rusznak & Peebles, 2002). However, some food allergies appear to be lifelong, e.g. nuts and seafood (Sampson, 1999).

Drugs

Drugs are a major cause of anaphylaxis. Approximately 62% of admissions to hospital with anaphylaxis are caused by therapeutic drugs (Sheikh & Alves, 2000). In the US drugs account for approximately 17% of all anaphylactic reactions, of which 5% are fatal (Weiler, 1999 and Yocum et al., 1999).

Parenteral administration of drugs is associated with a higher risk of anaphylaxis than oral administration (Joint Taskforce on Practice Parameters, American Academy of Allergy, Asthma and Immunology and the Joint Council of Allergy, Asthma and Immunology, 1998 and Beck & Burks, 1999). Drugs used in irrigation can also cause anaphylaxis (Antevil et al., 2003).

Penicillin and its derivatives account for the majority of drug-induced anaphylaxis episodes (Zull, 1999 and Peebles & Adkinson, 2000). In the US penicillin is responsible for 75% of drug-induced anaphylactic reactions (Joint Taskforce on Practice Parameters, American Academy of Allergy, Asthma and Immunology and the Joint Council of Allergy, Asthma and Immunology, 1998).

Aspirin and non-steroidal anti-inflammatory drugs (NSAID) are recognised causes of anaphylaxis (Zull, 1999). In one review they were the cause in 50% of drug-induced episodes of anaphylaxis and in 10% of the overall total episodes (Kemp et al., 1995). A study undertaken in The Netherlands found that in a 15-year period 76 cases of NSAID-induced anaphylaxis were reported (van Puijenbroek et al., 2002). Fatalities are possible (Sen et al., 2001).

In children, drugs are rarely the cause of anaphylaxis. However, when a drug is identified as the cause, it is usually the penicillin group of antibiotics (Alves & Sheikh, 2001).

It is worth noting that in reported suspected reactions to penicillin (mild non-specific rash to anaphylaxis) based on the clinical history alone, only 20% are confirmed to be genuine (Ponvert et al., 1999). As it is not possible to confirm or exclude penicillin allergy from the clinical history alone, all patients should be referred to an allergist (Clark & Ewan, 2002).

Latex

Latex is an important cause of occupational allergy (Yunginger, 1999).

Latex-induced anaphylaxis is on the increase, probably because of the enormous increase in the use of latex gloves in the healthcare environment (Ewan, 2000a), as part of a regime for universal precautions against blood-borne infections (Bird, 1996).

Latex allergy is common among healthcare workers who routinely use latex gloves: studies suggest the incidence could be as high as 10% (Hunt, 1993). In the USA alone, the numbers of pairs of gloves supplied to hospitals rose from 785 million in 1980 to 4.5 billion in 1992 (Allergy UK, 2003b). Some people who are sensitive to latex react to latex particles shed by gloves or their lining powder (Allergy UK, 2003b).

Other groups who are particularly prone to latex allergy include:

- Those with existing atopy, perhaps because of the increased opportunity for sensitisation via eczematous skin (Bird, 1996)
- Women who have repeated vaginal examinations (Cox & Grady, 2002 and Shingai et al., 2002)
- Children and young adults with abnormalities of the spine – frequent exposure to latex through urinary catheterisations (Bird, 1996)
- Those who have frequent operative procedures – latex-induced anaphylaxis has been reported during surgery (Leynadier et al., 1988) and radiographic procedures (Sussman et al., 1992).

Popular cosmetic hair alterations use latex-containing bonding glue to attach hair to the scalp. Cogen and Beezhold (2002) reported a case of a 37-year-old woman who developed anaphylaxis following repeated exposure to hair bonding glue. Tests demonstrated that hair-bonding glue contains significantly high concentrations of soluble latex antigen, which could cause anaphylaxis without mucosal contact. This reported cause of anaphylaxis is not an isolated incident (Wakelin, 2002).

Latex allergy is usually slower in onset (30 minutes) because the allergen is absorbed through the skin (Ewan, 2000a). Reactions are provoked

Table 2.1   Common sources of latex

Hospital	Other
Gloves	Balloons
Catheter	Rubber bands
Syringes	Carpet backing
Vials	Lycra in clothes
Masks	Furniture filling
Many disposable items	Elastic in clothing

Source: Latex Allergy Newsletter, Allergy UK, 2003b

by the absorption of latex through the skin or mucosal surfaces; latex can also cause respiratory symptoms when inhaled (Clark & Nasser, 2001). Bernardini et al. (2002) reported a case of anaphylaxis to latex following the ingestion of a cream-filled doughnut contaminated with latex.

Latex-induced anaphylaxis in children is rare, often only associated with those who require frequent surgical procedures and/or indwelling urinary catheters (Kelly et al., 1994). There have been reported cases of anaphylaxis resulting from contact with plastic balls in a play pit (Fiocchi et al., 2001).

Several recent reports support the existence of reactions to latex pacifiers (dummies) in infants; in one, an atopic 2-month-old baby experienced repeated stridor on exposure to a latex nipple while feeding (Freishtat & Goepp, 2002).

Avoidance involves the use of synthetic gloves with high-risk patients and the use of low-allergen, powder-free latex gloves in areas of frequent use to minimise topical and airborne exposures (Woods et al., 1997). Wynn (1998) reported one hospital in the USA that has endeavoured to become totally latex free. Avoiding latex may result in a decrease in IgE antibodies in latex-sensitised patients (Reider et al., 2002). Common sources of latex are detailed in Table 2.1.

Insect venom

Insects that sting are members of the order Hymenoptera (Reisman, 1992). They can be divided up into families including the Apidae (e.g. honey bee, bumble bee) and the Vespidae (e.g. wasp, yellowjacket) (Reisman, 1992). In the UK, most reactions are caused by wasp stings (Ewan, 2000b). Interestingly, those allergic to wasp venom are rarely allergic to bee venom (Ewan, 2000b). People allergic to bee venom are generally those who have been stung frequently by bees, e.g. beekeepers, their families, and possibly their neighbours (Ewan, 2000b).

Anaphylaxis following an insect sting is not uncommon (Reisman, 1992), the incidence in the general population being between 0.5 and 4% (Clark & Nasser, 2001). Interestingly, more than 90% of stings occur in the under-20-years age group, whereas 93% of deaths from insect stings occur in the over-20s (Zull, 1999). Symptoms usually start 10–20 minutes after the sting (Reisman, 1992).

Insect stings can be fatal (Volcheck, 2002). Oropharyngeal stings are particularly dangerous, owing to the potential to develop life-threatening airway obstruction via localised swelling (Smoley, 2002).

In the UK, Coroners' data suggest that on average there are four deaths annually attributed to bee or wasp stings (Ewan, 2000b), and in the USA approximately 50 deaths (Smoley, 2002 and Ditto, 2002). However, these are certainly underestimates, because venom-induced anaphylaxis is not always recognised as the cause of death – unexplained deaths at the poolside or on golf courses, as well as those attributed to cardiac causes, may be caused by unrecognised anaphylaxis (Ditto, 2002).

In children, insect (bee and wasp) venom-induced anaphylaxis is rare (Pumphrey & Stanworth, 1996). Moreover, children with existing atopy (asthma/rhinitis) do not have an increased risk of systemic complications (Novembre et al., 1998 and Settipane et al., 1980). In addition, children who develop a venom allergy (skin reactions only) often recover spontaneously without treatment (Valentine et al., 1990).

Following venom-induced anaphylaxis, it is impossible to predict the severity of the reaction to the next sting; in one large study the severity of the reaction was less in 45% of cases, the same in 43% of cases and worse in 12% (Settipane et al., 1980). Specific immunotherapy for the venom is effective at preventing a future systemic reaction (Yunginger, 1998).

Exercise

Exercise is an underdiagnosed cause of anaphylaxis (Zull, 1999). Since its first description in 1979 (Maulitz et al., 1979), it has become an increasingly recognised and reported phenomenon (Casale et al., 1986, Hough & Dec, 1994, Dutau et al., 2001 and Castells et al., 2003). Adams (2002) reported a case of exercise-induced anaphylaxis in a marathon runner. Cold-dependent exercised-induced anaphylaxis has been reported (Ii et al., 2002), but is rare (Briner, 1995).

The syndrome often requires both exercise and the ingestion of particular foods (Edwards & Johnston, 1997). Most individuals are unaware of concomitant food sensitivity because ingestion does not cause symptoms unless they exercise within 2–6 hours (Atkinson & Kaliner, 1992).

Although food-induced reactions may occur frequently with exercise-induced anaphylaxis, related factors are often present (Castells et al., 2003). A carefully taken history is particularly important when making a diagnosis (Perkins & Keith, 2002). It is more common in those with a history, or a family history, of atopy and in those who exercise in hot, humid conditions (Briner, 1995). Some foods, particularly shellfish, alcohol, fruit, wheat, celery and milk, are more likely to exacerbate exercise-induced anaphylaxis, though the mechanism is not known (Shadick et al., 1999). In some cases no specific food appears to be the problem but any meal followed by exercise can cause symptoms. Children with exercise-induced anaphylaxis often have a history of urticaria and sensitisation to inhalant or food allergens (Clark & Ewan, 2002).

The frequency of attacks may be reduced if exercise following meals is avoided (Novembre et al., 1998). It is recommended to stop exercising immediately a rash begins to appear, and to always exercise with a friend who is carrying an adrenaline (epinephrine) emergency kit (Zull, 1999).

The occurrence of reactions seems to stabilise or diminish over time, and improvement seems to be associated with exercise modification and avoidance of environmental and food precipitants (Rusznak & Peebles, 2002).

Radiocontrast media

The incidence of anaphylaxis in patients who receive radiocontrast media is reported to be 1%, and that of death 0.001–0.009% (Vervloet & Durham, 2000). In the US it is the third commonest cause of anaphylaxis-related death (Zull, 1999). Radiocontrast media can cause mast cell degranulation by a direct non-IgE-mediated mechanism (Clark & Nasser, 2001).

The risk of reactions can be minimised by using newer (and safer) radiocontrast media (Vervloet & Durham, 2000) and by administering a steroid and an antihistamine prior to the procedure (Bush & Swanson, 1991).

The management of anaphylaxis associated with IV contrast media is discussed in detail in Chapter 6.

Vaccinations

Vaccination-induced anaphylaxis is uncommon (Rusznak & Peebles, 2002). The Department of Health (1996) reported that:

- During a 3-year period from 1992 to 1995, 55 million doses of vaccines were supplied to hospitals and GPs. During the same period the Medicines Control Agency, through their Yellow Card reporting scheme (see pages 103–4), received 87 reports of anaphylactic reactions in patients of all ages following immunisations. No deaths were reported.
- During the national Measles and Rubella Immunisation Campaign in November 1994, approximately 8 million children from 5 to 16 years of age (5–18 in Scotland) were immunised; 81 cases of anaphylaxis were reported (1:100 000), slightly more common in those over 9 years of age and in girls. No deaths were reported.

Although there have been reported cases of anaphylaxis to the measles–mumps–rubella (MMR) vaccine (Pool et al., 2002), they are rare and most commonly occur in children not allergic to eggs (Khakoo & Lack, 2000). Children with a history of anaphylaxis have been safely immunised with MMR (Patja et al., 2001).

Until recently, egg allergy was considered to be a contraindication to receiving vaccines which had been produced in embryonated eggs (James et al., 1998). However, the administration of these vaccines to patients with egg allergy is now considered safe (Rusznak & Peebles, 2002).

The most likely cause of the anaphylaxis is another component of the vaccine, e.g. gelatin or neomycin (Patja et al., 2001). In fact, 25% of patients with reported anaphylaxis following the MMR vaccine seem to have hyper-sensitivity to the gelatin (heat stabiliser) component (Pool et al., 2002).

Gelatin

Gelatin is an important cause of anaphylaxis (Kelso, 1999). It is used in foods, vaccines and medications (Nakayama et al., 1999). Reported cases of vaccine-induced anaphylaxis were caused by the presence of gelatin in the vaccine (Sakaguchi et al., 1996). Anaphylactic reactions to gelatin-containing rectal suppositories have also been reported (Sakaguchi & Inouye, 2001).

Idiopathic

Approximately one-third of all anaphylactic reactions have no identifiable cause (Kemp et al., 1995). When no eliciting factors can be identified, the term 'idiopathic anaphylaxis' is used; it is therefore a diagnosis of exclusion, which can only be made after careful allergy history taking and diagnosis involving in vitro tests (Ring & Darsow, 2002). First described in the late 1970s (Bacal et al., 1978), it is indistinguishable from allergen-specific episodes, except that there is a higher incidence of upper airway angioedema (Zull, 1999).

In one study of 81 patients with idiopathic anaphylaxis:

- 68% were female
- 48% had a notable prevalence of atopic diseases
- 20% had a food allergy
- 15% had episodes of anaphylaxis with an identifiable cause
- only 9% had vascular involvement (Tejedor et al., 2002).

Causes of anaphylaxis associated with anaesthesia

Suspected Anaphylactic Reactions Associated with Anaesthesia, published by the Association of Anaesthetists of Great Britain and Ireland and British Society of Allergy and Clinical Immunology (1995), provides guidance on the management of suspected anaphylaxis associated with anaesthesia. Incidence figures for anaphylaxis episodes associated with anaesthesia quoted in this document include the following:

- Between 1991 and 1994, 90 (four fatal) suspected anaphylaxis episodes associated with anaesthesia were reported to the Medicines Control Agency.
- In France the incidence of anaphylaxis in anaesthesia is estimated to be 1 in 6000, and in Australia between 1 in 10 000 and 1 in 20 000.
- In the UK the estimated number of anaphylaxis episodes per year is between 175 and 1000.
- It is more common in women.

Muscle relaxants cause anaphylaxis in 1 in 4500 general anaesthetics (Vervloet & Durham, 2000): rocuronium is commonly implicated (Rose & Fisher, 2001). Anaesthetic drug-induced anaphylaxis is usually seen during induction of anaesthesia.

Anaphylaxis due to latex is becoming increasingly common, particularly in patients undergoing abdominal and gynaecological surgery; the reaction usually begins 30–60 minutes after the start of the procedure (in contrast to drugs).

Chlorhexidine is also a recognised cause of anaphylaxis during anaesthesia; this is a skin disinfectant commonly used prior to surgery and invasive procedures, and symptoms usually start about 20–40 minutes after application (Garvey et al., 2001).

A recent 2-year survey in France of anaphylaxis episodes ($n = 477$) during anaesthesia found that the majority of the reactions were in females (72%), and causes included:

- Muscle relaxants (69%) – particularly rocuronium
- Latex (12.1%)
- Antibiotics (8.0%) (Laxenaire & Mertes, 2001).

Chapter summary

Although the exact prevalence of anaphylaxis in the general population is unknown, the incidence is steadily rising. Causes of anaphylaxis include therapeutic drugs, food, insect stings, contrast media and latex. Anaphylaxis episodes associated with anaesthesia are not uncommon.

Diagnosing anaphylaxis

Introduction

Diagnosing anaphylaxis can be difficult because of the lack of a consistent clinical picture (Project Team of the Resuscitation Council (UK), 2002). Many conditions, including vasovagal episodes (following parenteral injections) and panic attacks, have been misdiagnosed as anaphylaxis, and patients with genuine anaphylaxis do not always receive the appropriate therapy (AHA & ILCOR, 2000). It is therefore important to ensure that an accurate and reliable diagnosis of anaphylaxis is made so that the most appropriate treatment can then be administered (after the event investigations, e.g. skin prick tests, can help to identify the causative allergen and confirm the diagnosis of anaphylaxis).

The aim of this chapter is to provide an overview to the diagnosing of anaphylaxis.

Chapter objectives

At the end of the chapter the reader will be able to:

- Outline the difficulties of diagnosing anaphylaxis
- List the clinical features of anaphylaxis

- Discuss the importance of history and examination
- Outline the immediate investigations that can be made
- Discuss the importance of differential diagnosis.

Difficulties with diagnosing anaphylaxis

There can be difficulties with diagnosing anaphylaxis because:

- The onset and specific signs and symptoms of anaphylaxis can vary considerably, depending on the sensitivity of the person and the route, quantity and rate of exposure to the allergen (Bochner & Lichtenstein, 1991).
- No single clinical finding is pathognomonic (AHA & ILCOR, 2000).
- Some of the clinical features that may be associated with anaphylaxis are similar or identical to manifestations of other local or systemic diseases (Bird, 1996).

The following will assist with diagnosing anaphylaxis:

- Knowledge of clinical features
- Full history and clinical examination
- Key investigations
- Differential diagnosis.

Investigations to identify the causative allergen and confirm the diagnosis of anaphylaxis retrospectively during later assessment and management are discussed in Chapter 8.

Clinical features

The onset of anaphylaxis is usually sudden, occurring within minutes of exposure to the allergen (Ewan, 2000a). Occasionally the onset may be delayed by a few hours and even persist for longer than 24 hours (Fisher, 1986). Reactions have even been reported days after exposure to an allergen (Reisman & Livingston, 1989).

The process of anaphylaxis can be slow, rapid or (unusually) biphasic (Chamberlain, 2001). Usually, the symptoms of anaphylaxis peak within minutes (Zull, 1999). Approximately 5% of patients experience a recurrence of anaphylaxis within 24 hours of the ending of the first reaction (Douglas et al., 1994). Mortality has particularly been associated with this reappearance of symptoms (Yunginger et al., 1988).

Anaphylaxis can vary in severity (Chamberlain, 2001). Generally, the severity of the reaction is proportional to the rapidity of its onset (Zull, 1999). Anaphylaxis that develops within 30 minutes is the most lethal (Joint Taskforce on Practice Parameters, American Academy of Allergy, Asthma and Immunology and the Joint Council of Allergy, Asthma and Immunology (1998) and Beck & Burks (1999)).

The presenting clinical features of anaphylaxis will depend on the route of exposure and the dose of the allergen, the severity and the systems affected. The possible presenting clinical features of anaphylaxis are listed in Table 3.1.

Table 3.1 Clinical features of anaphylaxis (depend on the route of exposure of the allergen, severity and systems affected)

Respiratory	Cardiovascular	Cutaneous	Gastrointestinal	Neurological
Dyspnoea	Tachycardia	Urticaria	Nausea and vomiting	Agitation
Rhinitis	Hypotension	Pallor	Abdominal cramps	Apprehension
Rhinorrhoea		Flushing	Diarrhoea	Altered levels of consciousness
Hoarseness		Angioedema		Feeling of impending doom
Stridor				
Wheeze				

Clinical assessment of the patient

An accurate clinical assessment of the patient is essential; in each case a full history and examination should be undertaken as soon as circumstances allow (Project Team of the Resuscitation Council (UK), 2001).

It is important to establish whether the patient has any known allergies or if there is a previous history of anaphylaxis. The events immediately prior to the onset of the reaction are particularly important. The patient may be wearing a MedicAlert bracelet, which could provide the practitioner with valuable information (see page 91).

Examination of the patient involves a rapid assessment of airway, breathing, circulation, cerebral function and gastrointestinal function, together with observation of the skin.

> The condition of the skin, heart rate, blood pressure, upper airways and chest auscultation require particular attention (Project Team of the Resuscitation Council (UK), 2002).

Assessment of airway and breathing

Assessment of airway and breathing involves evaluating the work of breathing, the efficacy of breathing and the adequacy of ventilation.

Work of breathing

Signs of increased work of breathing include a rise in respiratory rate, noisy respirations and accessory muscle use (Jevon & Ewens, 2002):

• **Tachypnoea:** often the first manifestation of respiratory distress; if hyperventilation is present this may indicate that the patient is having a panic attack

- **Stridor:** 'croaking' respirations, more pronounced during inspiration, could indicate laryngeal oedema (sometimes it may be preceded by hoarseness, or the patient may complain of a 'lump in the throat')
- **Wheeze:** a noisy musical sound caused by turbulent flow of air through narrowed bronchi and bronchioles which is more pronounced on expiration, indicating bronchospasm.

Efficacy of breathing
- Evaluate air entry by looking, listening and feeling for signs of breathing, auscultating the chest and observing chest movement. In particular check for the presence of a wheeze. A silent chest is an ominous sign (Jevon & Ewens, 2002).
- Commence pulse oximetry – 'normal' oxygen saturation should be >95% (Jevon & Ewens, 2002).
- (Arterial blood gas analysis).

Adequacy of ventilation
Assess the heart rate, skin colour and the patient's mental status. Signs of hypoxaemia include:

- Tachycardia (severe hypoxia can cause bradycardia)
- Pallor initially; central cyanosis is a late and often preterminal sign
- Agitation or impaired conscious level.

Measurement of peak expiratory flow rate
Measurement of peak expiratory flow rate (PEFR) (Fig. 3.1) is a simple test to ascertain the severity of bronchospasm in a patient with suspected anaphylaxis (Project Team of the Resuscitation Council (UK), 2002). The

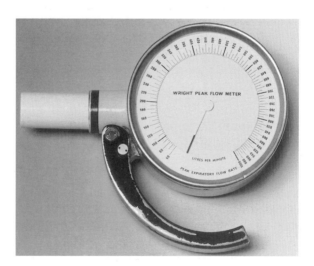

Fig. 3.1   A peak flow meter

normal peak flow is 400–700 litres/min and 300–500 litres/min in adult men and adult women respectively (Jevon et al., 2000).

Assessment of circulation

Pulses

Tachycardia, although non-specific, is an important sign of anaphylaxis. A rapid, weak, thready pulse and a discrepancy in the volume between central and distal pulses may be indicative of anaphylactic shock.

Blood pressure

Measurement of the blood pressure is paramount. Hypotension may be indicative of anaphylactic shock.

Peripheral perfusion

Poor peripheral perfusion, a sign of shock, is characterised by cool peripheries, skin mottling, pallor, cyanosis and delayed capillary refill (>2 s). Assess the capillary refill as follows:

- Raise the extremity, e.g. digit, slightly higher than the level of the heart (this will ensure the assessment of arteriolar capillary and not venous stasis refill).
- Blanch the digit for 5 s, then release. A delayed capillary refill (>2 s) may be indicative of anaphylactic shock (Jevon & Ewens, 2002).

Assessment of cerebral function

Assessment of conscious level can be carried out using the AVPU method, a simple, rapid and effective neurological scoring system which quantifies the response to stimulation and assesses conscious level (American College of Surgeons, 1997). It is ideal in the emergency situation when a rapid assessment of conscious level is required. AVPU stands for:

Alert
Responsive to Verbal stimulation
Responsive to Painful stimulation
Unresponsive.

Clinical signs of poor cerebral perfusion include a deterioration in conscious level, confusion, agitation and lethargy (Jevon & Ewens, 2002). Syncope, light-headedness or faintness can be associated with anaphylaxis.

Observation of the skin

In anaphylaxis, the skin colour usually changes (Project Team of the Resuscitation Council (UK), 2002). Possible changes include urticaria (Figs 3.2 and 3.3), flushing, pallor and angioedema. (NB: Severe hypotension can preclude these signs.)

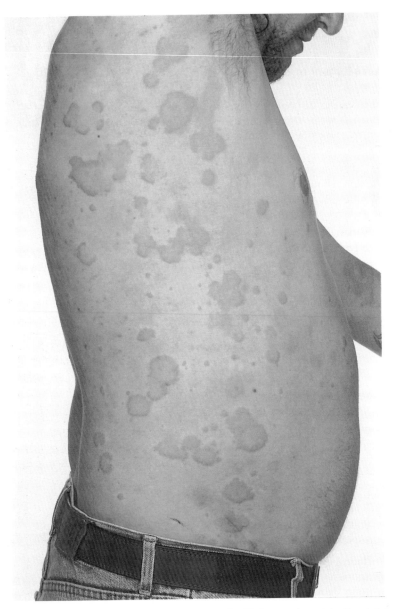

Fig. 3.2 Urticaria (The author is grateful to Dr M Bazza, Associate Specialist, Dermatology, Manor Hospital, Walsall, for his assistance)

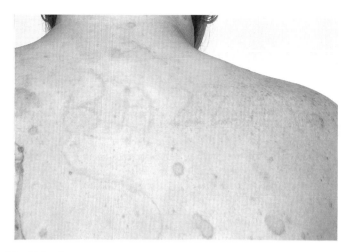

Fig. 3.3   Urticaria

Investigations

The only useful investigation that is available at the time of the reaction is the determination of serum tryptase (Ewan, 2000a). Tryptase is released from mast cells during anaphylaxis. It has a half-life of 60–90 minutes. The test is considered to be a highly specific and sensitive test for anaphylaxis (Fisher, 1997). It can also be used to help diagnose anaphylaxis retrospectively (Schwartz et al., 1994), even from postmortem specimens (Yunginger et al., 1991 and Fisher & Baldo, 1993). Although serum measurements of specific IgE antibody can be helpful, they do require careful interpretation.

Both of these blood tests can be undertaken on 10 mL of clotted blood, ideally taken 45–60 minutes – but no later than 6 hours – after the reaction (Project Team of the Resuscitation Council (UK), 2002). The use of blood tests should be encouraged because the future management of the patient can be helped by increased diagnostic certainty (Project Team of the Resuscitation Council (UK), 2002).

Serum histamine levels are raised during anaphylaxis. However, the serum half-life of histamine is very short, making detection difficult even in symptomatic periods (Tierney et al., 2002).

Importance of differential diagnosis

Several of the clinical features of anaphylaxis are either similar or identical to manifestations of other local or systemic diseases. In fact, many conditions have been misdiagnosed as anaphylaxis (AHA & ILCOR, 2000). Accurate clinical assessment is therefore important because the management of some of these other conditions may differ significantly from that of anaphylaxis (Bird, 1996).

Infection-induced upper airway obstruction

Although the clinical features of an infection-induced upper airway obstruction, e.g. croup and epiglottitis, may be similar to angioedema of the larynx and supraglottic region, the presence of pyrexia, pain and trismus would indicate infection (Zull, 1999).

Panic attacks and vasovagal episodes

It can be very difficult to distinguish between anaphylaxis, panic attacks and vasovagal episodes – all three can occur following an immunisation procedure (Resuscitation Council (UK), 2000). However, although some of the presenting signs and symptoms may be similar, there are some important differences:

- **Panic attack:** can lead to hyperventilation, an anxiety-related erythematous rash and tachycardia; usually no hypotension, pallor, wheeze, angioedema and urticaria
- **Vasovagal episode:** can lead to collapse, syncope, bradycardia and hypotension; usually no urticaria, angioedema, tachycardia or dyspnoea.

Hereditary angioedema

Hereditary angioedema or C1 inhibitor deficiency is a rare condition, characterised by acute upper airway compromise, gastrointestinal symptoms or angioedema of the skin (Zull, 1999). However asthma and urticaria are not present (Bird, 1996). First line treatment (if available) is with 1000 units of C1-inh concentrate which is source and product screened for transmissible viruses. Adrenaline (epinephrine), antihistamines and steroids are **not** considered to be effective (Agostini & Cicardi, 1992 and Waytes et al., 1996).

Angioedema due to ACE inhibitor therapy

Angioedema of the tongue, oropharynx and larynx due to angiotensin-converting enzyme (ACE) inhibitor therapy occurs in 1:1000 patients and can be life-threatening (Zull, 1999). It usually manifests within 2 weeks of the commencement of therapy, though any time interval is possible (Roberts & Wuerz, 1991). Although the optimum medical management of this form of angioedema is unclear, aggressive early airway management is essential.

Scombroid fish poisoning

This often develops within 30 minutes of eating spoiled tuna, mackerel or dolphin; it usually manifests as palpitations, flushing, urticaria, nausea, vomiting, diarrhoea and headache, and is treated with antihistamines. The syndrome is self-limiting (Gellert et al., 1992).

Systemic mastocytosis and carcinoid syndrome

Systemic mastocytosis and carcinoid syndrome are rare disorders that are characterised by mediator release (Bird, 1996), producing episodes of flushing, urticaria and hypotension, occasionally precipitated by alcohol (Horan et al., 1991). Stings or opioid drugs may cause non-allergic anaphylaxis in patients with mastocytosis.

Circulatory shock

The presence of circulatory shock is a common clinical finding in anaphylaxis. However, there are many other causes of circulatory shock:

- **Loss of circulating volume (hypovolaemic shock):** causes include haemorrhaging, burns, severe vomiting and diarrhoea, and it can be a complication of intestinal obstruction
- **Cardiac pump failure (cardiogenic shock):** causes include myocardial infarction, cardiac arrhythmias and myocarditis
- **Mechanical obstruction to cardiac filling and cardiac output (obstructive shock):** causes include pulmonary embolism, tension pneumothorax and cardiac tamponade
- **Increased intravascular space caused by dilation of the systemic vasculature (distributive shock):** causes include sepsis and neurogenic (and anaphylaxis) (source: Jevon & Ewens, 2002).

In a patient with shock of unknown cause there should be a high index of suspicion for anaphylaxis, particularly if there is no evidence of hypovolaemia, sepsis or cardiac failure (Schwartz et al., 1995a).

Systemic capillary leak syndrome

Systemic capillary leak syndrome is characterised by shock and generalised oedema (Zull, 1999). The only effective treatment is volume replacement (Barnadas et al., 1995).

Monosodium glutamate symptom complex

Monosodium glutamate symptom complex ('Chinese restaurant syndrome') is characterised by flushing and bronchospasm (Zull, 1999). It can be distinguished from anaphylaxis by the absence of urticaria and angioedema and the presence of headache, chest pain and burning or numbness in the upper trunk, face and neck (Raiten et al., 1995).

Serum sickness

Serum sickness is a delayed allergic reaction, often associated with bee stings (Reisman, 1992). Characterised by urticaria, it is differentiated by the presence of pyrexia, joint pains and lymphadenopathy (Zull, 1999).

Munchausen or hysterical anaphylaxis

Sometimes patients feign stridor and respiratory distress (Snyder & Weiss, 1989): this is referred to as Munchausen or hysterical anaphylaxis (Zull, 1999). Munchausen anaphylaxis is not always hysterical; it can result from self-injection or self-exposure to a known trigger (Hendrix et al., 1981). Nevertheless, standard treatment is recommended unless indirect laryngoscopy is normal (Snyder & Weiss, 1989).

Chapter summary

The patient or witnesses to the onset of the symptoms should be asked about known allergies. What the patient was doing prior to the event may give important clues to help distinguish anaphylaxis from the other conditions listed below. Was the patient eating or exercising, was the patient stung, had they recently started new medication, had they complained about itching or a rash?

A carefully taken history is paramount if an accurate diagnosis of anaphylaxis is to be made. Knowledge of the events preceding the reaction can provide vital clues to the causative allergen. In later assessment and management (Chapter 8), tests and investigations may help to identify the causative allergen and provide a certain diagnosis of anaphylaxis.

Chapter 4

Management of anaphylaxis in adults

Introduction

'The management of anaphylaxis includes early recognition, anticipation of deterioration, and aggressive support of airway, oxygenation, ventilation, and circulation' (AHA & ILCOR, 2000).

Consensus guidelines for the emergency medical treatment of anaphylaxis in adults by first medical responders and in the community are available (Project Team of the Resuscitation Council (UK), 2002).

The aim of this chapter is to help the reader to understand the management of anaphylaxis in adults.

Chapter objectives

At the end of the chapter the reader will be able to:

- Outline the background to the publication of the consensus guidelines
- Discuss the emergency medical treatment of anaphylaxis in adults by the first medical responder
- Discuss the emergency medical treatment of anaphylaxis in adults in the community
- List the special circumstances that require treatment modification
- Discuss post-anaphylaxis management.

Background to the publication of the consensus guidelines

The consensus guidelines *Emergency Medical Treatment of Anaphylactic Reactions* provided a broad consensus on the appropriate emergency management of anaphylaxis by first medical responders, who were unlikely to have expert knowledge or specialist interest (Project Team of the Resuscitation Council (UK), 1999). The guidelines were not intended to replace existing advice on the management of anaphylaxis in specific circumstances:

- During anaesthesia (Association of Anaesthetists of Great Britain and Ireland and British Society of Allergy and Clinical Immunology, 1995)
- Procedures involving injection of contrast medium (Board of Faculty of Clinical Radiology, Royal College of Radiologists, 1996) (see Chapter 6)
- Immunisation programmes (Department of Health, 1996)
- Treatment by paramedics (Statement from the Resuscitation Council (UK) and the Joint Royal Colleges Ambulance Service Liaison Committee, 1997).

Why they were needed

The guidelines were originally published at a time when anaphylaxis was considered to be poorly managed, varying recommendations had been made concerning its management, and adrenaline (epinephrine) was greatly underused (Project Team of the Resuscitation Council (UK), 1999).

Evidence base

No definitive clinical trials had been undertaken to provide an unequivocal evidence base for the management of anaphylaxis; in addition, it is unlikely that such evidence will be forthcoming (Project Team of the Resuscitation Council (UK), 1999). However, considerable experience on the management of anaphylaxis does exist. This experience was integrated through the broad membership of the Project Team.

Project Team

The Project Team was convened under the aegis of the Resuscitation Council (UK) to draw up the guidelines. Chaired by Douglas Chamberlain, it comprised representatives from the:

- Royal College of General Practitioners
- Association of Anaesthetists
- Royal College of Paediatrics and Child Health
- Royal College of Radiologists
- Anaphylaxis Campaign
- British Society for Allergy and Clinical Immunology
- British National Formulary
- Royal College of Pathologists
- British Association of Emergency Medicine.

Safety considerations

The Project Team acknowledged that the diagnosis of anaphylaxis can sometimes be difficult, particularly in children. Therefore, when writing the guidelines, the inevitability of some diagnostic errors was taken into account and particular emphasis placed on the importance of safety (Project Team of the Resuscitation Council (UK), 1999).

Feedback following publication

Although the guidelines were generally well received, the following concerns were raised:

- Adherence to the new guidelines would be difficult for community nurses because they did not have access to the drugs mentioned, except adrenaline (epinephrine)
- Paediatric drug doses of adrenaline (epinephrine), particularly with the recommendation to use twofold dilution for the lowest dose
- Doses of adrenaline (epinephrine) recommended in the guidelines differed from those recommended in the *British National Formulary* (Project Team of the Resuscitation Council (UK), 2001).

Revision of guidelines

The guidelines were revised, taking into account the concerns raised. There were now four algorithms:

- Treatment algorithm for the management of anaphylaxis in adults by the first medical responder
- Treatment algorithm for the management of anaphylaxis in children by the first medical responder

- Treatment algorithm for the management of anaphylaxis in adults in the community
- Treatment algorithm for the management of anaphylaxis in children in the community.

The current guidelines can be accessed on the Resuscitation Council (UK) website: www.resus.org.uk (Project Team of the Resuscitation Council (UK), 2002).

Emergency medical treatment of anaphylaxis in adults by first medical responders

The approach to the treatment of anaphylaxis is difficult to standardise because aetiology, clinical presentation (including severity and course) and organ involvement vary widely (AHA & ILCOR, 2000). The algorithm in Figure 4.1 provides a structural and systematic approach, and summarises the current recommendations for the management of anaphylaxis by first medical responders.

Early recognition of the signs and symptoms

Early intervention is critical to the successful management of anaphylaxis (Rusznak & Peebles, 2002). It is therefore essential to recognise the signs and symptoms of anaphylaxis promptly (Table 4.1). Take a history, undertake a clinical assessment, and monitor the patient's vital signs (see pages 21–23). Diagnosing anaphylaxis was discussed in detail in Chapter 3.

Expert help

As soon as anaphylaxis is suspected summon expert help, following local protocols. Ideally this should include an experienced anaesthetist (Cox &

Table 4.1 Symptoms and signs in allergic reaction (Advanced Life Support Group, 2001)

	Symptoms	Signs
Mild	Burning sensation in mouth Itching of lips, mouth, throat Feeling of warmth Nausea Abdominal pain	Urticarial rash Angioedema Conjunctivitis
Moderate (mild+)	Coughing/wheezing Loose bowel motions Sweating Irritability	Bronchospasm Tachycardia Pallor
Severe (Moderate+)	Difficulty breathing Collapse Vomiting Uncontrolled defecation	Severe bronchospasm Laryngeal oedema Shock Respiratory arrest, Cardiac arrest

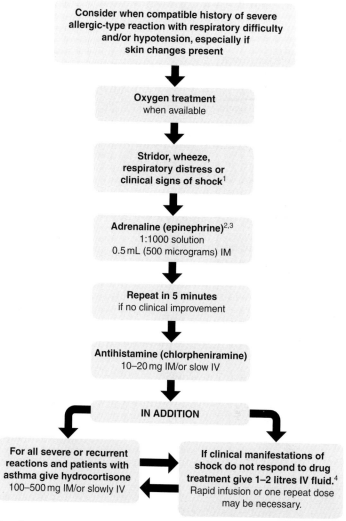

Fig. 4.1 Management of anaphylaxis in adults by the first medical responder (from, Update on the emergency medical treatment of anaphylactic reactions for community nurses. Project Team of the Resuscitation Council (UK). Resuscitation 2001; 48: 341–3). Reproduced with permission of Aurum Pharmaceuticals in association with the Resuscitation Council (UK)

Grady, 2002). An ENT surgeon may also be required if the airway is severely compromised, possibly necessitating an emergency tracheostomy.

Resuscitation equipment

The necessary resuscitation equipment, including more aggressive and invasive methods of life support such as intubation and tracheotomy, should be summoned (Bochner & Lichtenstein, 1991).

Preventing further exposure to the allergen

If possible, prevent further administration and absorption of the allergen (Bochner & Lichtenstein, 1991). For example:

- **Bee sting:** scrape any insect parts off the skin (Visscher et al., 1996) – do not squeeze them, as this allegedly increases envenomation (AHA & ILCOR, 2000)
- **IV infusion:** discontinue
- **Topical exposure:** wash the skin thoroughly (Zull, 1999)
- **Ingested allergen:** consider charcoal administration.

Patient position

Recline the patient into a comfortable position (Project Team of the Resuscitation Council (UK), 2002). If the patient is hypotensive, lie him or her flat and elevate the legs (unless respiratory distress is exacerbated). NB: There have been reported cases of patients with anaphylactic shock who, following a change to a more upright posture, have developed cardiac arrest (Pumphrey, 2003).

Oxygen

> Administer 10–15 L of oxygen per minute, via a face mask with a non-return valve and oxygen reservoir bag.

Oxygen is an important adjunctive therapy (Rusznak & Peebles, 2002) and high flow rates are recommended (AHA & ILCOR, 2000). Administer 10–15 L of oxygen per minute, via a face mask with a non-return valve and oxygen reservoir bag. This will result in the delivery of approximately 85% oxygen (Jevon, 2002). Instigate pulse oximetry (Fig. 4.2) and ECG monitoring (ECG signs of myocardial ischaemia commonly occur in anaphylactic shock, but not in anaphylactic asphyxia).

Adrenaline (epinephrine)

> Adrenaline (epinephrine) is the most important drug in severe anaphylaxis (Fisher, 1995).

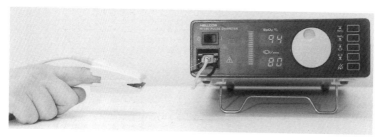

Fig. 4.2   Pulse oximetry and ECG monitoring (with permission from Blackwell Science)

An adrenoceptor agonist, adrenaline (epinephrine) acts on both α receptors and β receptors (Clark & Ewan, 2002):

- **α Receptor stimulation:** causes peripheral vasoconstriction, which will help to increase the blood pressure and reduce angioedema of the skin and mucous membranes (Zull, 1999)
- **β Receptor stimulation:** causes bronchodilation, increases the force of myocardial contraction and inhibits the further release of chemical mediators, e.g. histamine, from mast cells (Drugs & Therapeutic Bulletin, 2003).

Adrenaline (epinephrine) is currently available in a variety of formats (Fig. 4.3). As well as being available in the traditional ampoule format, it is also available in a prefilled syringe, although care should be taken to ensure the correct dose is administered.

Administer adrenaline (epinephrine) if there is stridor, wheeze, respiratory distress or clinical features of shock (Fisher, 1995 and the Project Team of the Resuscitation Council (UK), 2002). It is almost always effective (Ewan, 2000a) when administered promptly (Patel et al., 1994 and Zull, 1999).

> Indications for adrenaline (epinephrine): stridor, wheeze, respiratory distress or clinical features of shock (Project Team of the Resuscitation Council (UK), 2002)

The recommended dose and route of administration are as follows:

- **Dose:** 500 µg (0.5 mL of 1:1000 solution); this can be repeated after 5 minutes if there is no improvement or if deterioration has occurred, particularly if the patient's conscious level becomes, or remains, impaired in the presence of hypotension (Project Team of the Resuscitation Council (UK), 2001). Several doses may be required (British Medical Association & Royal Pharmaceutical Society of Great Britain, 2001)
- **Route:** IM into the thigh (Simons et al., 2001 and Sicherer, 2003).

The site of injection significantly affects the peak plasma concentrations of adrenaline (epinephrine) (Rusznak & Peebles, 2002). The IM route is recommended, preferably into the thigh and not the arm (Simons et al., 2001). Although the subcutaneous adrenaline (epinephrine) route has

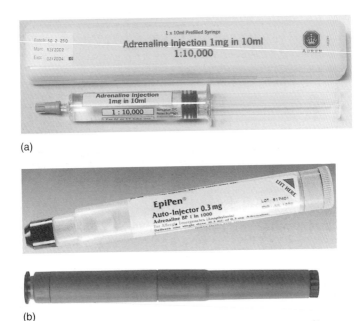

(a)

(b)

Fig. 4.3 (a) Adrenaline (epinephrine) (Reproduced by permission of Aurum Pharmaceuticals) and (b) autoinjector devices (EpiPen, reproduced by permission of ALK-Abello UK Ltd; Anapen, reproduced by permission of Celltech) in a pre-filled syringe format

previously been advocated by some authorities (Drugs & Therapeutic Bulletin, 1994) it is no longer the route of choice, particularly if the patient is in shock, because absorption and achievement of therapeutic plasma concentrations can be significantly delayed (Simons et al., 1998).

The IM route is relatively safe and adverse effects are rare (Project Team of the Resuscitation Council (UK), 2002). Reported side-effects include nausea, tremor, anxiety, palpitations, a rise in blood pressure and headache (Simons et al., 2002a). The only reported case of myocardial infarction was in a patient with multiple risk factors for coronary heart disease (Saff et al., 1993). In fact, it is not always possible to be certain whether complications are allergen or adrenaline (epinephrine) induced (Project Team of the Resuscitation Council (UK), 2002). In any case, the benefits of adrenaline (epinephrine) far outweigh the risks (Rusznak & Peebles, 2002).

The more hazardous IV route is occasionally used, particularly if the patient is in profound shock which is judged to be immediately life-threatening, or in certain situations, e.g. anaesthesia (Ewan, 2000a), and only if IV access is available (AHA & ILCOR, 2000). The IV route of administration 'should usually be reserved for medically qualified personnel who have experience of it, who know that it must be administered with extreme care, and who are aware of the hazards associated with its use' (Project Team

---

Case study   Dangers of IV adrenaline (epinephrine)

Johnston et al. (2003) commented on the case of a 40-year-old woman who had presented to A&E with generalised urticaria and angioedema, 30 minutes after taking pseudoephedrine and diphenhydramine for acute sinusitis. She had a history of mild asthma, but no cardiac disease. She had no hypotension or respiratory distress.

Adrenaline (epinephrine) 1 mL 1:1000, chlorpheniramine 10 mg and hydro-cortisone 100 mg were administered, all IV. The patient subsequently developed pulseless ventricular tachycardia and required cardiopulmonary resuscitation. She did make a full recovery.

Johnston and her colleagues comment that adrenaline (epinephrine) was inappropriately administered. Both the dose administered and the strength used for IV administration contravene current guidelines.

---

of the Resuscitation Council (UK), 2002). The risks of IV administration of adrenaline (epinephrine) include hypotension, cardiac arrhythmias and myocardial infarction (Barach et al., 1984, Zull, 1999 and Johnston et al., 2003).

In order to minimise complications following IV administration the 1:10 000 solution, i.e. 100 μg/mL (and not the 1:1000 solution) of adrenaline (epinephrine) should be used and administration should be slow, with increments (Ewan, 2000). The patient's ECG should be closely monitored.

Although inhaled adrenaline (epinephrine) is effective in cases of mild to moderate laryngeal oedema, it would not be given if IM adrenaline (epinephrine) has already been administered and it is not a substitute for IM adrenaline (epinephrine) (Ewan, 2000a).

In animal studies, administering adrenaline (epinephrine) sublingually in tablet form has been shown to be effective in achieving peak plasma concentrations (Gu et al., 2002). Absorption studies in humans are required before this non-invasive method of administering adrenaline (epinephrine) in the first-aid setting can be considered (Gu et al., 2002).

Very occasionally adrenaline (epinephrine) will fail to reverse the clinical manifestation of anaphylaxis, particularly in delayed reactions or in patients on β-blocker therapy; other measures, especially volume replacement therapy, will then assume greater importance (Project Team of the Resuscitation Council (UK), 2002).

Antihistamine

An antihistamine (H_1 blocker) such as chlorphenamine (Fig. 4.4) should be administered to help counteract the histamine-mediated vasodilation (Project Team of the Resuscitation Council (UK), 2002). It will also relieve the cutaneous manifestations of urticaria (Tierney et al., 2002). The recommended dose for chlorphenamine is 10–20 mg, either IM or slow IV. If the latter route is used, care should be taken to avoid drug-induced hypotension.

Sometimes an H_2 blocker, e.g. cimetidine, is administered (Runge et al., 1992). Unlike H_1 blockers, H_2 blockers do not cause drowsiness (Moscati &

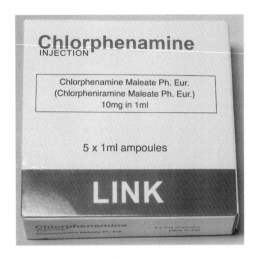

Fig. 4.4   An antihistamine (H_1 blocker)

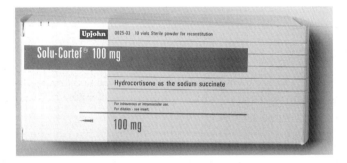

Fig. 4.5   A corticosteroid

Moore, 1990) or induce hypotension (Yarbrough et al., 1989). However, they can exacerbate bronchospasm (Zull, 1999).

Corticosteroid

A corticosteroid (Fig. 4.5) should be administered following severe anaphylactic reactions to help prevent late sequelae (Ewan, 2000a), particularly in asthmatics who have been on corticosteroid treatment previously, because they are at increased risk of severe or fatal anaphylaxis (Project Team of the Resuscitation Council (UK), 2002).

Although some authors are unenthusiastic about the use of hydrocortisone in anaphylaxis (Brown, 1998), the benefit of steroids in the management of status asthmaticus is well documented (Littenberg & Gluck, 1986). However, corticosteroids will not reverse airway obstruction or shock (Tierney et al., 2002).

The recommended dose of hydrocortisone is 100–500 mg either IM or by slow IV injection. Again, care should be taken to avoid inducing further hypotension.

The effects may not be evident until several hours following administration (Rusznak & Peebles, 2002).

Fluids

If severe hypotension fails to respond rapidly to drug therapy, fluids should be infused. A rapid infusion of 1–2 L may be required initially (Resuscitation Council (UK), 2000a). There is an ongoing debate as to whether to use a crystalloid or a colloid. Schierhout and Roberts (1998) recommend using a crystalloid because it is 'safer'; however, this has recently been challenged. The current guidelines still state that 'a crystalloid may be safer than a colloid' (Project Team of the Resuscitation Council (UK), 2002).

Inhaled β_2 agonist

An inhaled β_2 agonist can help to reverse bronchoconstriction (Rusznak & Peebles, 2002). Considered useful, it is indicated if bronchoconstriction is a prominent feature that is not responding to conventional treatment (Project Team of the Resuscitation Council (UK), 2002). If the patient is hypotensive, administer adrenaline (epinephrine) first, so as not to cause a further fall in blood pressure (AHA & ILCOR, 2000). Measurement of peak expiratory flow rate is a useful guide to the severity of the bronchospasm.

There have been some interesting case reports demonstrating the value of magnesium sulphate to reverse otherwise irreversible bronchospasm (Pumphrey & Nicholls, 2000).

Glucagon

Glucagon should be considered if adrenaline (epinephrine) is ineffective, particularly if the patient has been taking β-blockers (AHA & ILCOR, 2000). The recommended dose is 1–2 mg IV over 5 minutes (Zull, 1999).

Life-threatening airway obstruction

Of particular concern is the potential rapid progression to life-threatening airway obstruction and asphyxia. Angioedema of the uvula, tongue, soft palate or lips could indicate concomitant laryngeal oedema. The presence of hoarseness, dysphagia or a lump in the throat should be approached aggressively, rather than waiting for stridor and drooling to develop (Zull, 1999). The following should be noted:

- Undertake early elective tracheal intubation in patients with hoarseness, lingual oedema and posterior or oropharyngeal swelling (AHA & ILCOR, 2000).
- Undertake semielective (awake, sedated) tracheal intubation without paralysing agents if respiratory function deteriorates (AHA & ILCOR, 2000).

- If tracheal intubation is indicated, although the oral route is preferred for direct visualisation the presence of supraglottic angioedema may make this difficult: the nasal route may be a better alternative (Zull, 1999).
- If tracheal intubation fails, cricothyrotomy may need to be performed (Atkinson & Kaliner, 1992).
- If tracheal intubation is delayed, progressive stridor, severe dysphonia or aphonia, laryngeal oedema, significant angioedema and hypoxaemia can develop, making tracheal intubation and cricothyrotomy very difficult or even impossible (AHA & ILCOR, 2000). Moreover, attempts at tracheal intubation may compromise the airway further by increasing laryngeal oedema and causing bleeding into the oropharynx and narrow glottic opening (AHA & ILCOR, 2000).
- The use of a paralysing agent prior to attempted tracheal intubation can be hazardous. If tracheal intubation is unsuccessful, even bag/valve/mask ventilation may prove impossible if an effective seal between the mask and the patient's face cannot be secured because of facial oedema – spontaneous breathing will not be possible owing to the administration of a paralysing agent (AHA & ILCOR, 2000).

Clearly, it is important to recognise the early warning signs of potential airway compromise and act promptly before further deterioration occurs. If required, tracheal intubation should be performed at an early stage, preferably by an experienced anaesthetist.

Assessment and reassessment

It is most important to monitor the patient closely. This involves assessment and constant reassessment of the vital signs:

- Airway – patency
- Breathing – mechanics, efficacy and adequacy, pulse oximetry, peak expiratory flow rate
- Circulation – pulse rate, cardiac monitoring to detect cardiac arrhythmias, blood pressure
- Conscious level – AVPU (see page 23).

This monitoring is important not only to evaluate the effectiveness of the treatment, but also to identify whether the patient is deteriorating. The patency of the upper airway and the patient's haemodynamic status should be closely monitored because laryngeal oedema (causing asphyxia) and shock are the principal causes of death associated with anaphylaxis (Zull, 1999).

Psychological care

There is no doubt that suffering an anaphylactic episode is very frightening for the patient. It has been suggested that anxiety could possibly exacerbate the effects of such an episode (Lalli, 1980). Reassuring the patient is not only good practice but it also appears that it may help to limit the effects of anaphylaxis (Howatson-Jones, 2000).

Special circumstances that require treatment modification

β-Blockers

β-Blockers may increase the severity of an anaphylactic reaction and antagonise the effects of adrenaline (epinephrine) (Toogood, 1988). There is also limited evidence that they may increase the incidence of anaphylaxis (Toogood, 1988 and Hepner et al., 1990). In patients taking β-blockers who develop anaphylaxis:

- Higher doses of adrenaline (epinephrine) may be required (Tierney et al., 2002) (caution if patient hypertensive). NB: the fact that the patient has been on β_2-blocker therapy should not prevent the use of adrenaline (epinephrine) (Ewan, 2000a).
- Glucagon may be effective (AHA & ILCOR, 2000 and Tierney et al., 2002)
- Inhaled ipratropium may be particularly useful in the treatment of bronchospasm (AHA & ILCOR, 2000).

ACE inhibitors

Patients taking ACE inhibitors may suffer from a greater degree of hypotension because the renin–angiotensin-dependent compensatory mechanism is inhibited (Tierney et al., 2002).

Tricyclic antidepressants or monoamine oxidase inhibitors

An interaction between tricyclic antidepressants or monoamine oxidase inhibitors and adrenaline (epinephrine) can be potentially dangerous (Project Team of the Resuscitation Council (UK), 2002). Patients on either of these medications should therefore receive half the standard dose of adrenaline (epinephrine).

Cocaine

As cocaine sensitises the heart to adrenaline (epinephrine), the latter should not be administered if the patient has taken cocaine (Cregler, 1991).

Emergency medical treatment of anaphylaxis in adults in the community

The algorithm depicted in Figure 4.6 details the emergency medical treatment of anaphylaxis in adults in the community. The management is similar to what has just been described for first medical responders. The algorithm takes into account the probable limited facilities, equipment and drugs in the community setting and stresses the:

- Urgency of arranging hospital transfer
- Need to administer adrenaline (epinephrine) promptly if there is stridor, wheeze, respiratory stress or clinical features of shock.

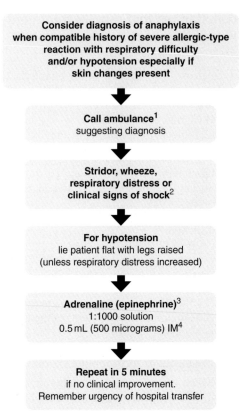

Consider diagnosis of anaphylaxis
when compatible history of severe allergic-type
reaction with respiratory difficulty
and/or hypotension especially if
skin changes present

Call ambulance[1]
suggesting diagnosis

Stridor, wheeze,
respiratory distress or
clinical signs of shock[2]

For hypotension
lie patient flat with legs raised
(unless respiratory distress increased)

Adrenaline (epinephrine)[3]
1:1000 solution
0.5 mL (500 micrograms) IM[4]

Repeat in 5 minutes
if no clinical improvement.
Remember urgency of hospital transfer

Notes [1]Ambulance will be equiped with oxygen, salbutamol, and fluids which may be used as adjunctive therapy. [2]If profound shock judged immediately life-threatening give CPR/ALS if necessary. [3]Half doses of adrenaline (epinephrine) may be safer for patients on amitriptyline, imipramine, or β-blocker. [4]If adults are treated with an Epipen, the 300 micrograms will usually be sufficient. A second dose may be required, but this should be considered ONLY if the patient's condition continues to deteriorate 5 minutes after the first dose. **NB** Remember the urgency of hospital transfer.

Fig. 4.6 Emergency medical treatment of anaphylaxis in adults in the community (from, Update on the emergency medical treatment of anaphylactic reactions for community nurses. Project Team of the Resuscitation Council (UK). Resuscitation 2001; 48: 241–3). Reproduced with permission from Aurum Pharmaceuticals in association with the Resuscitation Council (UK)

Post-anaphylaxis management

Both during and after an anaphylactic reaction it is most important to monitor the patient closely. This involves assessment and constant reassessment of the patient's vital signs. The patency of the upper airway and the patient's haemodynamic status should also be closely monitored.

Measurement of mast cell tryptase

Measurement of mast cell tryptase can help with the retrospective diagnosis of anaphylaxis (Schwartz et al., 1994). Serum tryptase levels are raised in the period immediately following an anaphylactic reaction (maximum level at 60 minutes). Serum levels of tryptase correlate linearly with the severity of the symptoms (Schwartz et al., 1995b).

Indications for admission

Biphasic reactions are not uncommon, particularly in patients who require higher doses of adrenaline (epinephrine) initially to control their symptoms (Brazil & MacNamara, 1998). Sometimes close monitoring for 8–24 hours will be required, particularly when the reaction:

- Is severe and slow in onset due to idiopathic anaphylaxis
- Occurs in a severe asthmatic
- Is complicated by a severe asthmatic attack
- Could be triggered again because further absorption of the allergen is possible (Project Team of the Resuscitation Council (UK), 2002).

Discharge of patient

All patients who are discharged following initial successful treatment for anaphylaxis must be informed of the risk of a second-phase reaction (Brazil & MacNamara, 1998). Consideration will need to be given to later assessment and management.

On-going assessment and management

The patient should be referred to an allergist, preferably one with experience in anaphylaxis (Bird, 1996 and Ewan, 2000a). The aim of later assessment is to identify/confirm the causative allergen where possible, and to educate the patient and general practitioner regarding future allergen avoidance and the appropriate management of any future episodes of anaphylaxis (Bird, 1996). The patient may also require an adrenaline (epinephrine) auto-injector device. On-going assessment and management are discussed in Chapter 8.

Chapter summary

This chapter has provided an overview to the consensus guidelines for the emergency treatment of anaphylactic reactions in adults by first medical responders and in the community. Anaphylaxis can be life-threatening. It is important to be able to recognise the clinical features of anaphylaxis and be familiar with the initial emergency management. If indicated, adrenaline (epinephrine) must be administered promptly.

Chapter 5

Management of anaphylaxis in children

Introduction

'Anaphylaxis can be life-threatening because of the rapid onset of airway compromise due to laryngeal oedema, breathing difficulties due to sudden severe bronchoconstriction and/or the development of shock due to acute vasodilation and fluid loss from the intravascular space caused by increased capillary permeability' (Advanced Life Support Group, 2001).

'The management of anaphylaxis includes early recognition, anticipation of deterioration, and aggressive support of airway, oxygenation, ventilation, and circulation' (AHA & ILCOR, 2000).

Consensus guidelines for the emergency medical treatment of anaphylaxis in children by first medical responders and in the community are available (Project Team of the Resuscitation Council (UK), 2002).

The aim of this chapter is to help the reader understand the management of anaphylaxis in children.

Chapter objectives

At the end of this chapter the reader will be able to:

- Discuss the important considerations when diagnosing anaphylaxis in children
- Discuss the emergency medical treatment of anaphylaxis in children by the first medical responder
- Discuss the emergency medical treatment of anaphylaxis in children in the community
- Discuss post-anaphylaxis management.

Important considerations when diagnosing anaphylaxis in children

The process of diagnosing anaphylaxis is discussed at length in Chapter 3. However, there are important considerations when diagnosing anaphylaxis in children:

- Recognising laryngeal oedema in children can be difficult; signs and symptoms include stridor, hoarseness, drooling or an alteration in voice pitch (Clark & Ewan, 2002).
- Respiratory distress (present in 79% of anaphylactic reactions) is more common than cardiovascular collapse (Novembre et al., 1998). In one study that analysed anaphylactic reactions to peanuts in children, severe respiratory distress occurred in 68% of reactions and hypotension in only 14.5% (all of which had respiratory distress as well) (Ewan, 1996).
- Anaphylaxis can be mistaken for acute severe asthma in children (Clark & Ewan, 2002). If a patient presents with 'asthma' but response to bronchodilators is poor, consider the possibility of anaphylaxis (Rainbow & Browne, 2002). In fact, the diagnosis of anaphylaxis is often overlooked in children with asthma. It has been recommended that children who have survived 'acute asphyxial asthma' should be screened for common allergens that are associated with asthma (Rainbow & Browne, 2002).
- Children with cardiovascular collapse often complain of feeling faint, look pale and have reduced muscle tone (Clark & Ewan, 2002).
- GI symptoms are common, e.g. dysphagia, nausea and vomiting, cramps and diarrhoea (Edwards & Johnston, 1997).
- There have been reported problems of diagnosing anaphylaxis in children (Project Team of the Resuscitation Council (UK), 2002). The lack of a consistent clinical picture can sometimes make an accurate diagnosis difficult. A detailed history and examination is essential as soon as possible, and a provisional diagnosis should be made based on the child's vital signs and clinical assessment.
- It is possible to mistake a panic attack, or hysteria following an injection, for anaphylaxis. A panic attack can lead to hyperventilation, an anxiety-related erythematous rash and tachycardia. However, there will be no hypotension, pallor, wheeze or urticarial rash (Project Team of the Resuscitation Council (UK), 2002).

Emergency medical treatment of anaphylaxis in children by first medical responders

As with adults, the approach to the treatment of anaphylaxis in children is difficult to standardise because aetiology, clinical presentation (including severity and course) and organ involvement vary widely (AHA & ILCOR, 2000). The algorithm in Figure 5.1 provides a structured and systematic approach. It summarises the current recommendations for the management of anaphylaxis in children by first medical responders.

Early recognition of the signs and symptoms

Early intervention is critical to the successful management of anaphylaxis (Rusznak & Peebles, 2002). It is therefore paramount to recognise the signs and symptoms of anaphylaxis promptly (Table 5.1). Diagnosing anaphylaxis is discussed in detail in Chapter 3.

Expert help

As soon as anaphylaxis is suspected summon expert help, following local protocols – this will usually be a paediatrician. If the child has a compromised airway, request anaesthetic and ENT help (Advanced Life Support Group, 2001). (In the out-of-hospital setting alert the Emergency Services.)

Resuscitation equipment

The necessary resuscitation equipment, including more aggressive and invasive methods of life support such as intubation and tracheotomy, should be summoned (Bochner & Lichtenstein, 1991). ECG monitoring should be commenced as soon as possible.

Preventing further exposure to the allergen

If possible, prevent further exposure to the allergen (Advanced Life Support Group, 2001).

Position child

The child will probably be very frightened. Help maintain a position of comfort (usually sitting), avoid unnecessary procedures and movement, and encourage the caregiver to stay and comfort the child (Edwards & Johnston, 1997). If the child develops shock, a supine position with the legs raised (unless respiratory distress is present) is recommended (Project Team of the Resuscitation Council (UK), 2002).

Oxygen

Administer high flow rates of oxygen (AHA & LCOR, 2000): ideally 10–15 L/min via a face mask with a non-return valve and oxygen reservoir bag (Fig. 5.2); this will result in the delivery of approximately 85% oxygen

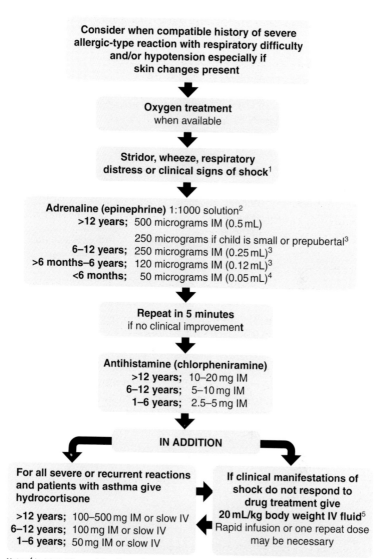

Consider when compatible history of severe allergic-type reaction with respiratory difficulty and/or hypotension especially if skin changes present

↓

Oxygen treatment
when available

↓

Stridor, wheeze, respiratory distress or clinical signs of shock[1]

↓

Adrenaline (epinephrine) 1:1000 solution[2]
>12 years; 500 micrograms IM (0.5 mL)

250 micrograms if child is small or prepubertal[3]
6–12 years; 250 micrograms IM (0.25 mL)[3]
>6 months–6 years; 120 micrograms IM (0.12 mL)[3]
<6 months; 50 micrograms IM (0.05 mL)[4]

↓

Repeat in 5 minutes
if no clinical improvement

↓

Antihistamine (chlorpheniramine)
>12 years; 10–20 mg IM
6–12 years; 5–10 mg IM
1–6 years; 2.5–5 mg IM

↓

IN ADDITION

For all severe or recurrent reactions and patients with asthma give hydrocortisone
>12 years; 100–500 mg IM or slow IV
6–12 years; 100 mg IM or slow IV
1–6 years; 50 mg IM or slow IV

If clinical manifestations of shock do not respond to drug treatment give
20 mL/kg body weight IV fluid[5]
Rapid infusion or one repeat dose may be necessary

Notes [1]An inhaled β_2-agonist such as salbutamol may be used as an adjunctive measure if bronchospasm is severe and does not respond rapidly to other treatment. [2]For profound shock judged immediately life-threatening give CPR/ALS if necessary. Consider slow IV adrenaline (epinephrine) 1:10 000 solution. This is hazardous and is recommended only for an experienced practitioner who can also obtain IV access without delay. **Note** the different strength of adrenaline (epinephrine) required for IV use. [3]For children who have been prescribed EpiPen, 150 micrograms can be given instead of 120 micrograms, and 300 micrograms can be given instead of 250 micrograms or 500 micrograms. [4]Absolute accuracy of the small dose is not essential. [5]A crystalloid may be safer than a colloid.

Fig. 5.1 Algorithm summarising the current recommendations for the management of anaphylaxis in children by first medical responders. (From, Update on the emergency medical treatment of anaphylactic reactions for first medical responders. Project Team of the Resuscitation Council (UK). Resuscitation 2001; 48: 241–3). Reproduced with permission of Aurum Pharmaceuticals in Association with the Resuscitation Council (UK)

Table 5.1 Symptoms and signs in allergic reaction (Advanced Life Support Group, 2001)

	Symptoms	Signs
Mild	Burning sensation in mouth Itching of lips, mouth, throat Feeling of warmth Nausea Abdominal pain	Urticarial rash Angio-oedema Conjunctivitis
Moderate (Mild+)	Coughing/wheezing Loose bowel motions Sweating Irritability	Bronchospasm Tachycardia Pallor
Severe (Moderate+)	Difficulty breathing Collapse Vomiting Uncontrolled defaecation	Severe bronchospasm Laryngeal oedema Shock Respiratory arrest Cardiac arrest

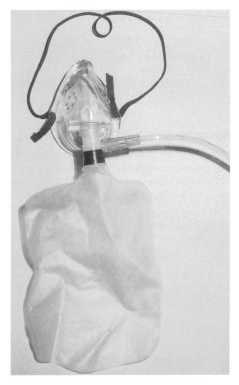

Fig. 5.2 An oxygen mask

to the child (Jevon, 2002). If the child is unable to tolerate the mask, ask the parents/caregiver to help, for example by holding the mask near the child's face. Pulse oximetry will help evaluate oxygenation (Edwards & Johnston, 1997).

Adrenaline (epinephrine)

Adrenaline (epinephrine) is the most important drug in severe anaphylaxis (Fisher, 1995), yet it is greatly underused (Clark & Ewan, 2002). It is almost always effective (Ewan, 2000a) when administered promptly (Patel et al., 1994 and Zull, 1999). Failure to administer adrenaline (epinephrine) may increase the likelihood of progression to cardiac arrest.

Administer adrenaline (epinephrine) if there is stridor, wheeze, respiratory distress or clinical features of shock (Fisher, 1995 and Project Team of the Resuscitation Council (UK), 2002). Using a 1:1000 solution $(100\,\mu g/0.1\,mL)$, the recommended dose of adrenaline (epinephrine) is related to the child's age:

- **>12 years:** $500\,\mu g$ IM $(0.5\,mL)$ $(250\,\mu g$ if the child is small or prepubertal)
- **6–12 years:** $250\,\mu g$ IM $(0.25\,mL)$
- **>6 months–6 years:** $120\,\mu g$ IM $(0.12\,mL)$
- **<6 months:** $50\,\mu g$ IM $(0.05\,mL)$ – absolute accuracy of this small dose is not essential (Project Team of the Resuscitation Council (UK), 2002).

One dose is usually sufficient (Wong et al., 1999). However, it should be repeated after 5 minutes if there is no clinical improvement (Project Team of the Resuscitation Council (UK), 2002). Sometimes several doses will be required (British Medical Association & Royal Pharmaceutical Society of Great Britain, 2001).

The IM route for the administration of adrenaline (epinephrine) is generally used as it is relatively safe and adverse effects are rare. The thigh is the preferred and recommended route (Simons et al., 2001 and Sicherer, 2003).

Administering adrenaline (epinephrine) intravenously is hazardous and may cause death (Pumphrey & Roberts, 2000). However, it should be considered if the child is in profound shock which is immediately life-threatening, or in certain situations, e.g. anaesthesia; it is therefore only recommended for experienced practitioners who can secure IV access quickly (Project Team of the Resuscitation Council (UK), 2002). To minimise the risk of complications of IV administration:

- Use the 1:10000 solution $(100\,\mu g/mL)$ of adrenaline (epinephrine); further dilution will increase its safety by reducing the risk of adverse effects (Brown, 1998)
- Administer slowly, with increments (Ewan, 2000a), closely monitoring the child's ECG.

Very occasionally adrenaline (epinephrine) will fail to reverse the clinical manifestation of anaphylaxis, despite repeated doses and fluid boluses. An infusion of adrenaline (epinephrine) may be life-saving: a dose of 0.1–5.0 µg/kg/min is recommended and the child's pulse and blood pressure must be closely monitored (Advanced Life Support Group, 2001).

If the child has laryngeal oedema, it is also recommended to administer nebulised adrenaline (epinephrine) 5 mL 1:1000 (Advanced Life Support Group, 2001).

Antihistamine

An antihistamine, e.g. chlorphenamine, should be used routinely in all anaphylactic reactions. Its use may be beneficial and is unlikely to be harmful (Project Team of the Resuscitation Council (UK), 2002). It will help counteract the histamine-mediated vasodilation and relieve the cutaneous manifestations of urticaria. Care should be taken to avoid drug-induced hypotension. The recommended dose of chlorphenamine is related to the child's age:

- **>12 years:** 10–20 mg IM or slow IV
- **6–12 years:** 5–10 mg IM or slow IV
- **1–6 years:** 2.5–5 mg IM or slow IV (Project Team of the Resuscitation Council (UK), 2002).

Cimetidine (H_2 blocker) may be useful in cases of refractory anaphylaxis (Edwards & Johnston, 1997).

Corticosteroid

A corticosteroid should be administered following severe anaphylactic reactions to help prevent late sequelae (Ewan, 2000a), particularly in asthmatics who have been on corticosteroid treatment previously because they are at increased risk of severe or fatal anaphylaxis (Project Team of the Resuscitation Council (UK), 2002). Care should be taken to avoid inducing further hypotension. The effects may not be evident until several hours after administration (Rusznak & Peebles, 2002). The recommended dose of hydrocortisone is related to the child's age:

- **>12 years:** 100–500 mg IM or slow IV
- **6–12 years:** 100 mg IM or slow IV
- **1–6 years:** 50 mg IM or slow IV.

Fluids

If severe hypotension fails to respond rapidly to drug therapy, fluids should be infused. A rapid infusion of 20 mL/kg is recommended (Advanced Life Support Group, 2001).

The crystalloid or colloid debate continues. Schierhout and Roberts (1998) recommend using a crystalloid because it is 'safer'; however, this has recently been challenged. One authoritative body recommends colloid (Advanced Life Support Group, 2001). The current guidelines still state that 'a crystalloid may be safer than a colloid' (Project Team of the Resuscitation Council (UK), 2002).

Inhaled β₂ agonist

An inhaled β_2 agonist may be used as an adjunctive measure if bronchospasm is severe and fails to respond rapidly to other treatment (Project Team of the Resuscitation Council (UK), 2002). Nebulised salbutamol 2.5–5 mg is recommended (Advanced Life Support Group, 2001). Measurement of peak expiratory flow rate is a useful guide to the severity of the bronchospasm.

Life-threatening airway obstruction

Clearly, it is important to recognise the early warning signs of potential airway compromise and act promptly before further deterioration occurs (see pages 21–22). If required, tracheal intubation should be performed at an early stage, preferably by an experienced paediatric anaesthetist.

Assessment and reassessment

It is most important to monitor the child closely. This involves assessment and constant reassessment of the vital signs:

- Airway – patency
- Breathing – mechanics, efficacy and adequacy, pulse oximetry, peak expiratory flow rate
- Circulation – pulse, heart rate, cardiac monitoring to detect cardiac arrhythmias, blood pressure, capillary refill
- Conscious level – AVPU (see page 23).

This is important not only to evaluate the effectiveness of the treatment, but also to identify whether the child is deteriorating. The patency of the upper airway and the patient's haemodynamic status should be closely monitored because laryngeal oedema (causing asphyxia) and shock are the principal causes of death associated with anaphylaxis (Zull, 1999).

Psychological care

There is no doubt that suffering an anaphylaxis episode is very frightening for the child. It has been suggested that anxiety could possibly exacerbate the effects of an anaphylaxis episode (Lalli, 1980). Reassuring the child is not only good practice but it also appears that it may help to limit the effects of anaphylaxis (Howatson-Jones, 2000). Allowing the parents/carer to stay with the child will also be helpful and reassuring for the child.

Emergency medical treatment of anaphylaxis in children in the community

The algorithm depicted in Figure 5.3 details the emergency medical treatment of anaphylaxis in children in the community. The management is similar to what has just been described for first medical responders. The

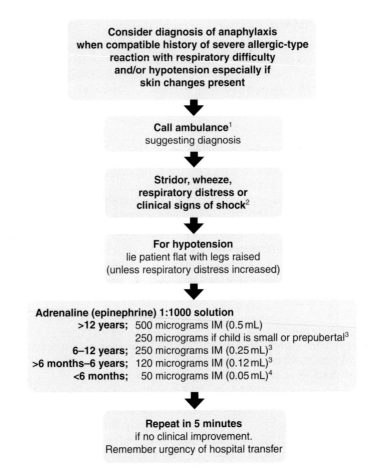

Consider diagnosis of anaphylaxis
when compatible history of severe allergic-type
reaction with respiratory difficulty
and/or hypotension especially if
skin changes present

⬇

Call ambulance[1]
suggesting diagnosis

⬇

Stridor, wheeze,
respiratory distress or
clinical signs of shock[2]

⬇

For hypotension
lie patient flat with legs raised
(unless respiratory distress increased)

⬇

Adrenaline (epinephrine) 1:1000 solution
>12 years; 500 micrograms IM (0.5 mL)
250 micrograms if child is small or prepubertal[3]
6–12 years; 250 micrograms IM (0.25 mL)[3]
>6 months–6 years; 120 micrograms IM (0.12 mL)[3]
<6 months; 50 micrograms IM (0.05 mL)[4]

⬇

Repeat in 5 minutes
if no clinical improvement.
Remember urgency of hospital transfer

Notes [1]Ambulance will be equipped with oxygen, salbutamol, and fluids which may be used as adjunctive therapy. [2]If profound shock judged immediately life-threatening give CPR/ALS if necessary. [3]For children who have been prescribed EpiPen, 150 micrograms can be given instead of 120 micrograms, and 300 micrograms can be given instead of 250 micrograms or 500 micrograms. [4]Absolute accuracy of the small dose is not essential.

Fig. 5.3 Algorithm detailing the emergency medical treatment of anaphylaxis in children in the community (from, Update on the emergency medical treatment of anaphylactic reactions for community nurses. Project Team of the Resuscitation Council (UK). Resuscitation 2001; 48: 341–3). Reproduced with permission of Aurum Pharmaceuticals in association with the Resuscitation Council (UK)

algorithm takes into account the probable limited facilities, equipment and drugs in the community setting and stresses:

- The urgency of arranging hospital transfer
- The need to administer adrenaline (epinephrine) promptly if there is stridor, wheeze, respiratory stress or clinical features of shock.

If the child has been prescribed an EpiPen Jnr or EpiPen or similar:

- EpiPen Jnr (150 μg) can be administered in children from 6 months to 6 years (instead of 120 μg)
- EpiPen (300 μg) can be administered in children over 6 years (instead of 250 μg or 500 μg) (Project Team of the Resuscitation Council (UK), 2002).

Inhaled adrenaline (epinephrine)

In the US, inhaled adrenaline (epinephrine) from a pressurised metered-dose inhaler is sometimes recommended as a non-invasive, user-friendly alternative to adrenaline (epinephrine) injection for out-of-hospital anaphylaxis (Simons et al., 2000). However, problems have been identified with this method. Research has demonstrated that, despite expert coaching, children are unable to inhale sufficient adrenaline (epinephrine) to increase plasma concentrations promptly and significantly because of the number of inhalations required and the bad taste of the inhalations (Simons et al., 2000). The authors of the study therefore urge caution in the recommending of adrenaline (epinephrine) inhalation as a substitute for the injection format for the out-of-hospital treatment of anaphylaxis in children.

Post-anaphylaxis management

Both during and after an anaphylactic reaction it is most important to monitor the child closely. This involves assessment and constant reassessment of the vital signs. The patency of the upper airway and the patient's haemodynamic status should also be closely monitored.

Measurement of mast cell tryptase

Measurement of mast cell tryptase can help with the retrospective diagnosis of anaphylaxis (Schwartz et al., 1994). Serum tryptase levels are raised in the period immediately following an anaphylactic reaction (maximum level at 60 minutes). Serum levels of tryptase correlate linearly with the severity of the symptoms (Schwartz et al., 1995b).

Indications for admission

Biphasic reactions are not uncommon, particularly if higher doses of adrenaline (epinephrine) are required initially to control the symptoms (Brazil & MacNamara, 1998). Sometimes close monitoring for 8–24 hours will be required, particularly when the reaction:

- Is severe and slow in onset due to idiopathic anaphylaxis
- Occurs in a severe asthmatic
- Is complicated by a severe asthmatic attack
- Could be triggered again because further absorption of the allergen is possible (Project Team of the Resuscitation Council (UK), 2002).

Discharge of child

If the child is discharged following initial successful treatment for ana-phylaxis, both the child (if appropriate) and the carer must be informed of the risk of a second-phase reaction. Consideration will need to be given to on-going assessment and management, including provision of an adrena-line (epinephrine) autoinjector device (and training).

On-going assessment and management

The child should ideally be referred to an allergist, preferably one with experience in anaphylaxis (Bird, 1996 and Ewan, 2000a). The cause of the anaphylaxis can be established by taking a structured allergy history and confirmed by the presence of specific IgE antibodies identified by skin prick tests or a specific challenge to confirm or exclude the diagnosis (Clark & Nasser, 2001). The child may also require an adrenaline (epinephrine) autoinjector device.

Advice should be given concerning allergen avoidance. This is backed up by educating the parents or carers and relevant school personnel (Ewan & Clark, 2001). Where appropriate this should include the effective administration of adrenaline (epinephrine). The wearing of a MedicAlert bracelet may be required. Later assessment and management are discussed in greater detail in Chapter 8. The management of anaphylaxis in the school environment is discussed in Chapter 9.

Chapter summary

This chapter has provided an overview to the consensus guidelines for the emergency treatment of anaphylactic reactions in children by first medical responders and in the community. Anaphylaxis can be life-threatening. It is important to be able to recognise the clinical features of anaphylaxis and be familiar with the initial emergency management. If indicated, adrena-line (epinephrine) must be administered promptly.

Chapter 6

Management of anaphylaxis caused by IV contrast media

Introduction

Contrast media are used in radiology departments to enhance the quality of images, facilitating diagnosis and treatment (Howatson-Jones, 2000). However, a recognised complication of IV contrast media is anaphylaxis, which can be fatal.

The Royal College of Radiologists has produced guidelines for the management of reactions to IV contrast media (Fig. 6.1) (Royal College of Radiologists, 1996). These guidelines are still valid and have not been superseded by the Consensus Guidelines (Project Team of the Resuscitation Council (UK), 2002). A separate chapter dealing with these guidelines would therefore be helpful.

The aim of the chapter is to help the reader understand the management of anaphylaxis to IV contrast media.

Chapter objectives

At the end of the chapter the reader will be able to:

• Discuss the incidence of anaphylaxis to IV contrast media
• Outline the essential points to consider when administering IV contrast media
• List the drugs that should be immediately available
• Outline the management of reactions to contrast media.

Incidence of anaphylaxis to IV contrast media

Anaphylaxis to IV contrast media can occur unexpectedly and may be life-threatening (Hong et al., 2002 and Nakamura et al., 2002). Cardiovascular collapse is the most common clinical finding (Shehadi, 1985).

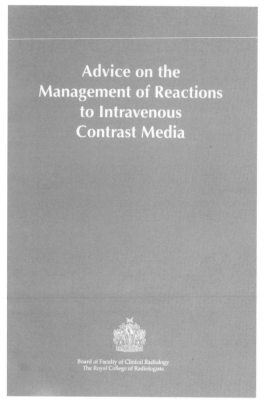

Fig. 6.1   Advice issued by the Royal College of Radiologists. Reproduced with permission

Although anaphylaxis following IV contrast media is reported to be rare, the incidence is thought to be increasing, probably because of the increased use of contrast media (Nakamura et al., 2002). The incidence is estimated to be 0.05% with ionic contrast media, but considerably less with non-ionic media (Royal College of Radiologists, 1996).

Following the recent adoption of non-ionic contrast media, the incidence of anaphylaxis will probably decrease. Using the smallest amount of contrast medium possible and low-molecular, non-ionic agents will also reduce the relative risk of reactions (Maddox, 2002).

In Japan, out of 163 363 procedures using non-ionic contrast media, only six (0.004%) anaphylaxis episodes and one fatality were reported (Katayama et al., 1990). In the US, in a 16-year period, 214 deaths attributable to IV contrast media were reported to the Food and Drug Administration (FDA); this equated to 2.1 fatalities per one million procedures (Lasser et al., 1997). Even though the incidence is low, as Shehadi (1985) pointed out, the patients were alive prior to the procedure and doubtless would have still been alive if it had not been undertaken.

The following risk factors for anaphylaxis episodes associated with IV contrast media have been proposed:

- History of allergy (Bush & Swanson, 1991 and Lieberman & Seigle, 1999)
- Asthma (Bush & Swanson, 1991 and Lieberman & Seigle, 1999)
- Age between 20 and 50 years (Bush & Swanson, 1991 and Lieberman & Seigle, 1999)
- Female gender (Lang et al., 1995)
- Cardiovascular disorder (Lang et al., 1993)
- Taking β-blockers (Lang et al., 1993).

Important considerations when administering IV contrast media

Important considerations when administering IV contrast media, as identified by the Royal College of Radiologists (1996) are as follows:

- Awareness of factors that increase risk is crucial. Any patients deemed to be at increased risk must receive a non-ionic agent, if any agent at all is received; see Royal College of Radiologists (1991) *Guidelines for Use of Low Osmolar Contrast Media*, Royal College of Radiologists, London.
- Each department should have a specific protocol for dealing with various reactions, which should be updated periodically. For children, the advice of local paediatric staff should be sought when considering the organisation of facilities. The advice of the local consultant anaesthetist designated to take responsibility for anaesthetic matters within the radiology department should be sought when formulating local policies.
- All personnel attending the patient should complete a basic resuscitation course on a regular basis. Those dealing with children should receive the appropriate training in paediatric resuscitation, which also needs to be regularly updated.
- The person who administers the contrast medium should have a basic medical history of the patient, particularly relating to risk factors, and be adequately trained in resuscitation procedures. Any person administering an intravenous contrast medium to children has a duty to be trained in paediatric resuscitation procedures.
- All persons involved in the daily running of the department in which the contrast medium is being administered should be aware of the site of resuscitation equipment. This should be immediately available: one trolley serving a unit scattered over several floors is not acceptable. Equipment and drugs should be regularly checked by a designated person (or persons) and recorded as checked. Resuscitation drugs for children should be stored separately in a box/trolley clearly labelled for use in children. Adult adrenaline (epinephrine) ampoules, clearly labelled, should be available in paediatric 'crash boxes' for the older, heavier child (>50 kg).
- Oxygen, with appropriate delivery systems for various ages, should be available in all rooms where intravenous contrast medium is

administered, particularly as oxygenation in compromised children is important.

- The weight of any child should be known and prominently displayed prior to the administration of intravenous contrast medium. A simple calculation of the relevant adrenaline (epinephrine) dose for the child should be made and recorded in a similarly prominent position.
- It is prudent to inject intravenous contrast medium through a needle which is securely taped and left in place for at least 15 minutes after administration of the medium, or until such time as it is considered safe to remove it if an adverse reaction has occurred. For children, ideally a 21–25 gauge cannula rather than a needle should be used. Depending on the severity of the reaction and the length of treatment required, an intravenous cannula should be inserted as soon as is practical in adults, and drugs administered through this rather than a needle, which carries the risk of cutting out.
- The patient should not be left alone following injection, particularly during the first 10 minutes. Serious reactions may sometimes be considerably delayed, and biphasic reactions are known to occur in up to 5% of patients.
- Contrast agents should not be injected in an isolated clinical setting. Non-ionic contrast medium should be used if a full cardiac arrest team is not available. Examinations requiring intravascular administration of contrast medium in children should only be undertaken in departments that have prompt access to a resuscitation team trained in paediatric resuscitation. All children should be injected with non-ionic contrast medium.

Points of emphasis with regard to drugs

The following points about drugs are reinforced:

- Antihistamines and hydrocortisone should never be mixed in the same syringe, as precipitation occurs.
- Corticosteroids are, quite correctly, considered as slow-acting drugs, with a lag time after injection of at least 6 hours. However, there is no doubt that they work very rapidly indeed when administered intravenously in severe bronchospasm and cardiovascular collapse, and should therefore not be withheld.
- Intravenous (IV) adrenaline (epinephrine) is potentially a dangerous drug associated with cardiac arrhythmias. It should not be used in minor reactions, but only in severe life-threatening bronchospasm, angioedema and/or cardiovascular collapse, when the potential benefits greatly outweigh the risks. Doses may have to be very high and may need to be repeated. Under normal circumstances adrenaline (epinephrine) should only be given by a member of the 'crash team', but every radiologist should be confident in the administration of intravenous or intramuscular/subcutaneous adrenaline (epinephrine), should the need arise, as it can be a potentially life-saving drug when administered early.
- Aminophylline is a drug that has fallen into disrepute in recent years as it may be associated with hypotension and collapse, and may only serve to exacerbate the clinical state of the patient.

Drugs that should be immediately available

The Royal College of Radiologists (1996) recommends that the following drugs should be immediately available where IV contrast agents are used:

- Chlorphenamine meleate
- Promethazine
- Hydrocortisone
- Atropine
- Salbutamol inhaler
- Salbutamol nebuliser
- Normal saline
- Gelofusine®
- Adrenaline (epinephrine), 1:10 000 and 1:1000.

Management of symptoms (Table 6.1)

Symptom complexes are listed in this section, together with their suggested management. Symptom complexes are placed in approximate ascending order of severity, but no attempt has been made to integrate symptomatology into a coherent aetiological scheme. Relevant information on the treatment of children is given under the information on management, in italics.

Please note that these guidelines date from 1996 and although they are undoubtedly helpful, it is important to be aware that some of the drug doses and interventions recommended do differ from current practice. However the guidelines can be used to help formulate local protocols.

Table 6.1

Symptom complex	Management
4.1 Nausea/vomiting	Reassure the patient Retain intravenous (IV) access and observe Antiemetics are rarely necessary
Mild scattered 'hives'/urticaria	Routine treatment is not necessary Retain IV access and observe If troublesome, administer an antihistamine, e.g. chlorphenamine maleate 10–20 mg (slow IV injection) *(paediatric dose: 0.2 mg/kg over 3–5 min)* or promethazine hydrochloride 25–50 mg (max. 100 mg) by slow IV injection *(not licensed for IV use in children)*
Severe generalised urticaria	Retain IV access and observe Administer IV antihistamines as above, with addition of IV hydrocortisone 100 mg *(paediatric dose: 4 mg/kg over 3–5 min)*
Mild wheeze	Retain IV access and observe

(Continued)

Table 6.1   (*Continued*)

	Give 100% oxygen at 10–15 L/min *(paediatric dose: 6–10 L/min)* by MC or Hudson mask (caution in hypercapnia) Give a β_2 agonist, for example salbutamol by nebuliser, 5 mg in 2 mL saline *(paediatric dose: 6 months to 5 years, 2.5 mg; >5 years, 5 mg)*. Repeat as necessary
Hypotension with bradycardia (vasovagal reaction/faint)	Raise the patient's feet Give 100% oxygen at 10–15 L/min by MC mask (caution with hypercapnia) *(paediatric dose: mask 6–10 L/min)* Establish 14–16 gauge cannula *(21–25 gauge in children)* Instigate ECG monitoring and oximetry Infuse rapid IV fluids (preferably colloid, e.g. Gelofusine® 10–15 mL/kg) to maintain blood pressure Inject IV atropine, 0.6 mg for bradycardia. Repeat at intervals of 5 min, up to 3 mg in total *(paediatric dose: 0.02 mg/kg, minimum dose 0.1 mg)* THE URGENT ADVICE OF AN ANAESTHETIST SHOULD BE REQUESTED
Hypotension alone, not vasovagal but no other signs of anaphylactoid reaction	Give 100% oxygen at 10–15 L/min by MC or Hudson mask *(paediatric dose: 6–10 L/min)* Infuse rapid IV fluids (colloid Gelofusine® 10–15 mL/kg) Establish blood pressure monitoring Instigate ECG monitoring and oximetry IF THERE IS NO RESPONSE AN ANAESTHETIST SHOULD BE SUMMONED FOR DIRECT SUPERVISION OF PRESSOR AGENTS, e.g. dobutamine 2.5–10 μg/kg/min, or dopamine 2–5 μg/kg/min *(paediatric patients should be managed by experts)*
Angioedema/urticaria/ bronchospasm/ hypotension leading to severe anaphylactoid reaction	Establish IV access 14–16 gauge cannula *(21–25 gauge in children)* Infuse rapid IV fluids (Gelofusine® 10–15 mL/kg) to maintain blood pressure Give 100% oxygen at 10–15 L/min by MC mask *(paediatric dose: 6–10 L/min)* Give a β_2 agonist, salbutamol by nebuliser, 5 mg in 2 mL saline *(paediatric dose: 6 months to 5 years, 2.5 mg; >5 years, 5 mg)*. DO NOT DELAY OTHER MEASURES TO SET THIS UP Inject IV hydrocortisone, 500 mg *(paediatric dose: 4 mg/kg, max. 200 mg)* Initiate ECG, blood pressure and oximetry monitoring If hypotension persists, administer IV adrenaline (epinephrine) at 0.5–1.0 mL of 1:10 000 *(paediatric dose: 0.1 mL/kg of 1:10 000, up to a limit of 1 mL)*

(*Continued*)

Table 6.1   (*Continued*)

Symptom complex	Management
	In severe cases, administer further aliquots of IV adrenaline (epinephrine) up to a total of 1 mg CALL FOR EMERGENCY ANAESTHETIC ADVICE
Unconscious/ unresponsive/ pulseless/ collapsed patient	SUMMON CRASH TEAM Institute standard cardiopulmonary resuscitation procedures as recommended by the Resuscitation Council (UK) (i) Basic life support: Establish airway, head tilt, chin lift Initiate ventilation, mouth to mouth Thump the precordium followed by external chest compression, 15 compressions to 2 breaths (*paediatric ratio: 5 compressions to 1 breath*) Continue uninterrupted until help arrives (ii) Advanced Life Support Establish IV fluids, 14–16 gauge cannula (*21–25 gauge in children*) Give 100% oxygen by bag/valve/mask ventilation Perform tracheal intubation Administer IV fluids at 10–15 mL/kg Instigate cardiac monitoring by ECG Perform DC cardioversion if in ventricular fibrillation (200 J, 200 J then 360 J) (*paediatric level: 2–4 J/kg*) Inject IV adrenaline (epinephrine) (1 mg = 10 mL of 1:10 000) (*paediatric dose: 0.1 mL/kg of 1:10 000*). Repeat adrenaline (epinephrine) as necessary (*at intervals of 15 min in children*) Consider administration of hydrocortisone/antihistamines during course of a successful resuscitation If no IV access give 0.3–1 mL of 1 in 1000 adrenaline (epinephrine) IM or SC (*paediatric dose: 0.01 mL/kg of 1:1000, IV dose may be given via interosseous cannula*) Consider endotracheal administration ADMIT PATIENT TO INTENSIVE CARE UNIT (ICU)
Seizure	May be the consequence of hypotension, and primary treatment should be as indicated in sections on previous page Give 100% oxygen, 10–15 L/min (*paediatric patient: 6–10 L/min*) by MC mask If seizure continues, anticonvulsant may be given, e.g. Diazemuls® IV 5–10 mg (*paediatric dose: Diazemuls® 0.2–0.3 mg/kg or diazepam emulsion 0.4 mg/kg*) initially, although higher doses may be needed Second-line drugs such as phenytoin may be required, but by this time the patient should be intubated and ventilated

Chapter summary

IV injection of contrast media is a major cause of anaphylaxis. Practitioners undertaking procedures involving the IV injection of contrast media must be familiar with the Royal College of Radiology's guidelines for the management of anaphylaxis. The recommended emergency drugs and resuscitation equipment must also be immediately available.

Chapter 7

Management of cardiac arrest associated with anaphylaxis

Introduction

The effective management of anaphylaxis involves early recognition and prompt aggressive treatment to prevent deterioration and avoid the dire situation of cardiac arrest. Even if cardiac arrest does develop, prompt aggressive therapy may still be successful (AHA & ILCOR, 2000).

However, prompt advanced life support (ALS) will be required if return of spontaneous circulation is to be achieved. ALS is the term used to describe the more specialised techniques employed to support breathing and circulation during cardiopulmonary resuscitation (CPR), as well as specific treatment used to try and restore cardiac output.

The European Resuscitation Council (ERC) ALS algorithms for the management of cardiac arrest in adults and children are universally applicable, though specific modifications are required to maximise the likelihood of success in a cardiac arrest associated with anaphylaxis. Although there is no data available on how CPR procedures should be modified for anaphylaxis, reasonable recommendations can be made based on experience with non-fatal cases (AHA & ILCOR, 2000).

The aim of this chapter is to provide a brief overview to the management of cardiac arrest associated with anaphylaxis.

Chapter objectives

At the end of the chapter the reader will be able to:

- Outline the ERC ALS algorithm
- Discuss the specific measures required
- Outline the ERC Paediatric ALS algorithm.

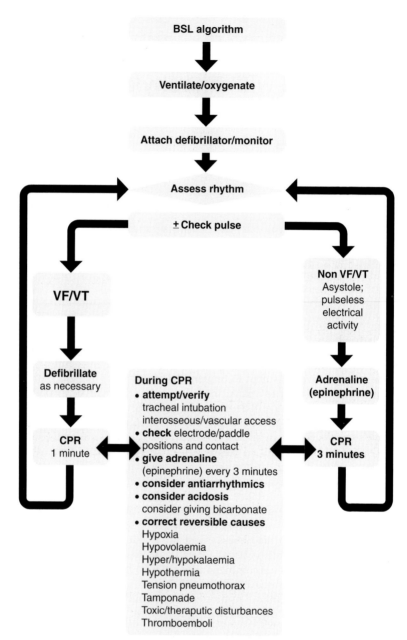

Fig. 7.1 ERC ALS algorithm (from 'European Resuscitation Council. Guidelines 2000 for Adult and Paediatric Basic Life Support and Advanced Life Support.' Resuscitation 2001; 48: 199–239)

ERC ALS algorithm

The ERC ALS algorithm (Fig. 7.1) is designed to be an *aide mémoire*, reminding the practitioner of the important aspects of assessment and treatment of cardiac arrest in adults. It is not designed to be comprehensive or limiting.

Entry into the algorithm depends on the events surrounding the event. If basic life support (BLS) is already in progress, this should continue while the cardiac monitor/defibrillator is attached. Cardiac monitoring provides the link between BLS and ALS. If the patient is already on a cardiac monitor, clinical and ECG detection of cardiac arrest will be almost simultaneous.

The presenting cardiac arrest arrhythmia can then be classified into one of two groups, depending whether or not defibrillation is required, i.e. VF/VT or non-VF/VT. The appropriate pathway in the algorithm is then followed.

Each step that follows in the algorithm assumes that the previous one has been unsuccessful. Looping the algorithm reinforces the concept of constant reassessment. Each step of the algorithm will now be discussed.

BLS algorithm if appropriate

Commence BLS, unless the patient is in VF/VT and can be defibrillated immediately. The ratio for BLS is two ventilations to 15 compressions.

Precordial thump if appropriate

Deliver a precordial thump (a sharp blow to the patient's sternum with a closed fist) if the cardiac arrest is witnessed or monitored, and a defibrillator is not immediately at hand (Resuscitation Council (UK), 2000).

Attach defibrillator/monitor

Ascertain the patient's ECG rhythm as soon as possible. Hopefully, in patients who develop anaphylaxis ECG monitoring will already have been established prior to collapse.

VF/VT pathway

VF/VT (Fig. 7.2) is thought to be uncommon in cardiac arrests associated with anaphylaxis (AHA & ILCOR, 2000), though it could complicate IV adrenaline (epinephrine) (Johnston et al., 2003). If VF/VT is identified, deliver up to three defibrillatory shocks (200 J, 200 J, 360 J or biphasic equivalent) as required (Resuscitation Council (UK), 2000a).

If defibrillation is unsuccessful, perform BLS for 1 minute (this will help preserve cerebral and myocardial function) and then reassess. Deliver a further sequence of up to three shocks of 360 J if required.

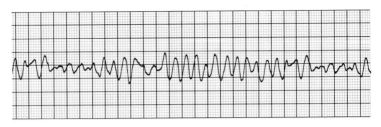

Fig. 7.2 VF/VT (uncommon in cardiac arrests associated with anaphylaxis) (Reproduced by permission of Medtronic Physio-Control Corp.)

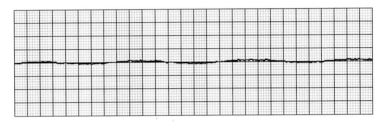

Fig. 7.3 Pulseless electrical activity (ischaemic changes likely to be present if anaphylactic shock prior to arrest)

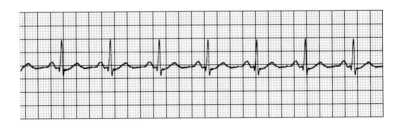

Fig. 7.4 Asystole

Non-VF/VT pathway

In a cardiac arrest associated with anaphylaxis the most likely presenting cardiac arrhythmia will be non-VF/VT, i.e. pulseless electrical activity (PEA) (Fig. 7.3) or asystole (Fig. 7.4) (AHA & ILCOR, 2000). If asystole is suspected, exclude other causes of a 'flat line' ECG trace by:

- Ensuring the ECG leads are correctly attached
- Ensuring the gain (ECG size) is correctly set
- Viewing the ECG through different leads, e.g. leads 1 and 2.

If asystole or PEA is confirmed, perform CPR for 3 minutes and then reassess the ECG trace and pulse (except if immediately following defibrillation: withhold drugs and perform CPR for 1 minute and then reassess the ECG trace and pulse; if asystole or PEA persists, perform CPR for a further 2 minutes and administer appropriate drugs).

During CPR

During CPR constant assessment and reassessment of airway, breathing and circulation is paramount:

- **Airway:** ensure a clear airway (see below)
- **Breathing:** ensure effective ventilation with 100% oxygen
- **Circulation:** monitor the ECG rhythm, checking for the presence of a pulse when appropriate; regularly check the accuracy of the ECG trace.

If it is not already, IV access should be secured with a wide-bore cannula. The chosen access will depend on the circumstances and expertise available. There are advantages and disadvantages of each route:

- **Peripheral route:** least invasive, has minimal complications and cannula insertion does not interfere with CPR. However, drugs can take 1–2 minutes to reach the central circulation (Khun et al., 1981). Following drug administration a 20 mL bolus of 0.9% normal saline and elevation of the limb are recommended (Emerman et al., 1990).
- **Central route:** can provide higher drug concentrations and has minimal circulation time. Unfortunately, it can be difficult to establish, can interrupt resuscitation, and complications can be catastrophic.

If IV access cannot be established the endobronchial route can be used for the administration of certain drugs, e.g. adrenaline (epinephrine) and atropine.

Doses of two to three times the standard IV dose, diluted with sterile water up to a total volume of 10–20 mL, are currently recommended when using this route (Resuscitation Council (UK), 2000a).

Drugs should be administered as appropriate:

- **Adrenaline (epinephrine):** routinely administered during CPR as it improves coronary and cerebral blood flow (Michael et al., 1984). The standard dose is 1 mg (10 mL of 1:10 000 solution) IV, repeated every 3 minutes. However, higher doses are recommended in a cardiac arrest associated with anaphylaxis (AHA & ILCOR, 2000) (see below).
- **Atropine:** antagonises the action of the vagus nerve and is recommended in asystole and PEA when the QRS rate is less than 60. The dose is 3 mg IV administered once only.
- **Amiodarone:** administered in refractory VF/VT (i.e. first three defibrillatory shocks unsuccessful). The initial dose is 300 mg IV; a further dose of 150 mg may be required.
- **Calcium:** indications include hypocalcaemia, hyperkalaemia and calcium channel blocker toxicity (unlikely to be used in a cardiac arrest associated with anaphylaxis); dose is 10 mL of 10% of calcium chloride IV.
- **Sodium bicarbonate:** rarely used because of its numerous adverse side-effects; may be considered if there is severe metabolic acidosis (pH <7.1

and base excess <10), hyperkalaemia or tricyclic overdose. The dose is 50 mmol IV (50 mL of 8.4% solution).
- **Magnesium sulphate:** indicated in refractory VF when there is suspicion of hypomagnesaemia. The dose is 4–8 mmol (2–4 mL of 50% magnesium sulphate) IV administered over 1–2 minutes. It may be repeated after 10–15 minutes.

Potential reversible causes of cardiopulmonary arrest

The search for, and treatment of, potential reversible causes of cardiac arrest is paramount, particularly when PEA is present. They can conveniently be classified into two groups for ease of memory – four 'Hs' and four 'Ts':

- *H*ypoxia
- *H*ypovolaemia
- *H*yperkalaemia/hypokalaemia and metabolic disorders
- *H*ypothermia
- *T*ension pneumothorax
- *T*amponade
- *T*hromboembolic or mechanical obstruction
- *T*oxic/therapeutic disturbances.

As tissue hypoxia, intravascular collapse and profound vasodilation are likely causes of cardiac arrest associated with anaphylaxis (AHA & ILCOR, 2000), treating these aggressively probably provides the optimum chance of patient survival. Attention to airway, oxygenation, ventilation and support of circulation is recommended (AHA & ILCOR, 2000).

Specific measures required

Airway, oxygenation and ventilation

Attempts should be made to secure the airway and provide adequate ventilation with 100% oxygen. However, the following difficulties may be encountered:

- Tracheal intubation may be impossible owing to upper airway swelling.
- Bag/valve/mask ventilation may be impossible because of difficulty in securing an adequate seal between the patient's face and the mask owing to the presence of angioedema.
- Cricothyrotomy may be difficult or indeed impossible because severe swelling can obliterate landmarks (AHA & ILCOR, 2000).

In a desperate situation, specific measures to secure the airway and support ventilation should be considered:

- Fibreoptic tracheal intubation
- Digital tracheal intubation: using the fingers insert a small tracheal tube (size 7 or less)
- Needle cricothyrotomy and transtracheal ventilation
- Cricothyrotomy as described by Simon and Brenner (1994) for a patient with massive swelling of the neck (AHA & ILCOR, 2000).

Circulation

Specific measures to support the circulation include:

- **High-dose adrenaline (epinephrine) IV:** high doses should be used without hesitation; a commonly used sequence is 1–3 mg IV (3 minutes), 3–5 mg IV (3 minutes) and then 4–10 μg/min (AHA & ILCOR, 2000).
- **Rapid volume expansion:** profound vasodilation leading to increased intravascular capacity can occur; large volumes of fluid should be administered quickly – 2–4 L of isotonic crystalloid are recommended.
- **Antihistamine IV:** although there are scarcely any data related to the value of administering antihistamines during CPR, it is very unlikely that additional harm could result (AHA & ILCOR, 2000). It would therefore be reasonable to administer chlorphenamine 10–20 mg IV.
- **Corticosteroid IV:** although corticosteroids are unlikely to have any effect during CPR, they may be helpful in the postresuscitation phase (AHA & ILCOR, 2000).

Prolonged CPR

Prolonged CPR may be necessary until the catastrophic effects of the anaphylactic reaction resolve.

ERC PALS algorithm

Paediatric advanced life support (PALS) is the term used to describe the more specialised techniques employed to support breathing and circulation during paediatric CPR, as well as specific treatment used to try and restore cardiac output. The ERC PALS algorithm (Fig. 7.5) is universally applicable, although specific modifications are required to maximise the likelihood of success in a cardiac arrest associated with anaphylaxis.

Most of the principles for managing a paediatric arrest associated with anaphylaxis are the same as those for an adult (discussed above). In particular, aggressive airway management and ventilation, adrenaline (epinephrine) and rapid fluid expansion are equally important. However, some key principles and differences need to be highlighted:

- **Initial priorities:** effective BLS and ventilation (Zideman & Spearpoint, 1999)
- **Compressions-to-ventilation ratio:** 5:1
- **IV access:** notoriously difficult in a paediatric arrest (Zideman & Spearpoint, 1999); the intraosseous route is recommended if IV access not established (Advanced Life Support Group, 2001)
- **Adrenaline (epinephrine):** the standard dose is 10 μg/kg (0.1 mL/kg of 1:10 000 solution), repeated every 3 minutes; in a cardiac arrest associated with anaphylaxis a higher dose (100 μg/kg) may be considered (Resuscitation Council (UK), 2000b)
- **Fluid boluses:** 20 mL/kg.

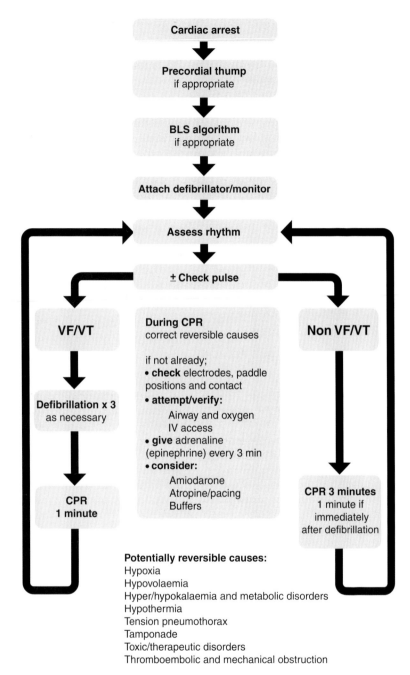

Fig. 7.5 The ERC PALS algorithm (from, European Resuscitation Council. Guidelines 2000 for Adult and Paediatric Basic Life Support and Advanced Life Support. Resuscitation 2001; 48: 199–239)

- **Documented hypoglycaemia:** administer glucose (American Academy of Pediatrics, 1997); the recommended dose is 0.5 g/kg dextrose (5 mL/kg of 10% dextrose) (Advanced Life Support Group, 2001).
- **Initial defibrillatory shocks:** 2 J/kg, 2 J/kg and 4 J/kg (or biphasic equivalent).

Chapter summary

Aggressive airway management and ventilation, high-dose adrenaline (epinephrine) and rapid volume expansion are key interventions in the management of cardiac arrest associated with anaphylaxis. Prolonged CPR may be required before return of spontaneous circulation is achieved. All CPR attempts should follow ERC guidelines.

Chapter 8

On-going assessment and management of anaphylaxis

Introduction

Regardless of the cause, patients who have experienced anaphylaxis should be referred to an allergist or clinical immunologist experienced in its management (Bird, 1996). The causative agent should be identified and advice given on avoidance to prevent further attacks (Ewan, 2000a). Ongoing support and education will be required and some patients will need to be equipped with an adrenaline (epinephrine) autoinjector device, together with full instructions in its use (Wynn et al., 1993 and Ewan, 2000a).

    The aim of this chapter is to provide an overview to the on-going assessment and management of anaphylaxis.

Chapter objectives

At the end of the chapter the reader will be able to:

- Discuss the importance of on-going assessment and management
- Discuss methods to identify the allergen
- Outline measures to avoid exposure to the allergen
- Describe the use of adrenaline (epinephrine) autoinjector devices
- Discuss the indications for desensitisation
- List the key action points to minimise the risk of anaphylaxis
- Describe the services offered by relevant charities.

Importance of on-going assessment and management

'The potential difficulty of correct diagnosis of an acute attack, combined with the need to assess accurately and exclude provoking factors for future anaphylaxis, highlights the importance of full assessment and design of future management strategies for all patients who have undergone previous severe allergic or anaphylactic events. Failure to undertake such assessments and implement management strategies has been a recurring theme in the audit of subsequent deaths from anaphylaxis' (Bird, 1996).

On-going assessment and appropriate management of the patient is therefore essential following an episode of anaphylaxis. The patient should be referred to an allergist, preferably one with expertise in anaphylaxis (Ewan, 2000a). At Cambridge, Ewan and her colleagues have demonstrated the value of an individual management plan for a severe allergy (Ewan & Clark, 2001). In a specialist allergy clinic for children with peanut allergy, they succeeded in reducing the number and severity of further anaphylaxis episodes.

Parham (2000) identified three distinct strategies that can be used to reduce the effects of allergic disease:

- **Prevention:** to modify a person's behaviour and environment, so that exposure to the allergen can be avoided
- **Pharmacological:** to use medications, e.g. antihistamines, corticosteroids and adrenaline (epinephrine), to minimise the impact of exposure to the allergen
- **Immunological:** to prevent the production of allergen-specific IgE – desensitisation can help achieve this (a therapeutic procedure in which an allergic person is exposed to increasing doses of allergen with the ultimate objective of inhibiting their hypersensitive response).

The causative allergen needs to be identified/confirmed and advice on avoidance provided. Information (patient and next-of-kin) relating to recognition of the signs and symptoms of a future anaphylaxis episode, together with how to deal with it, is paramount. Education regarding the use of an adrenaline (epinephrine) autoinjector device may also be required, together with the use of other medications, e.g. antihistamine. Desensitisation may be indicated in some situations. Advice and support from organisations such as the Anaphylaxis Campaign and Allergy UK can be very beneficial.

Methods to identify the causative allergen

Clinical history

The clinical history is extremely important (Fisher, 1995), as it is often possible to identify the allergen from this alone (Hendry, 2001). A detailed analysis of events surrounding the anaphylaxis reaction should be undertaken. Sometimes the cause is obvious from the history (Ewan, 2000a). Caution should be exercised when ascertaining a dietary history, because it can be notoriously inaccurate (Bock et al., 1988). Past medical history, including known allergies and previous episodes of anaphylaxis, is also important.

Skin-prick tests

Skin-prick tests, the most common investigation to assess sensitivity (Hendry, 2001), can be performed to support or discount a diagnosis of allergy (Kay, 2000). The ensuing release of histamine and other mediators produces a wheal and erythema, usually after 15 minutes (Hendry, 2001). The advantages and disadvantages of skin-prick tests are listed in Table 8.1.

Both positive (histamine 10 mg/mL) and negative (diluent) control solutions should be used (Kay, 2000). Aqueous solutions of a variety of allergens are currently available, including:

- Common inhaled allergens, e.g. dust mite, grass pollen
- Occupation allergens, e.g. latex, antibiotics
- Food allergens (Rusznak & Davies, 2000).

Durham (2000) recommends the following procedure for the skin-prick testing:

1. Explain the procedure to the patient.
2. Place a drop of the allergen solution on the skin of the forearm (Fig. 8.1).

Table 8.1 Skin-prick test: advantages and disadvantages (Rusznak & Davies, 2000)

Advantages	Disadvantages
Painless	Wheal and flare reaction can be suppressed by antihistamines
Minimal risk of side-effects	Test less reliable with food allergens
Informative to the patient	Itching causes slight discomfort
High patient compliance	Interpretation is difficult in patients with eczema or dermatographism
Can be undertaken in health centres	

3. Prick the skin through the allergen solution with a sterile lancet (Fig. 8.2) or 25 gauge (orange) needle, ensuring that a different needle is used for each allergen solution.
4. Remove the excess allergen solution from the skin using an absorbent paper tissue.
5. Evaluate the reaction after 15 minutes.

A reaction is generally deemed positive when a skin wheal in the positive control is >2 mm larger than that observed in the negative control (Kay, 2000). The result of the test should be interpreted in the light of the clinical history. Interpretation of skin-prick tests requires experience, because both false negative and false positive results can be observed (Bird, 1996). Anaphylactic reactions following skin-prick testing have been reported (Vanin et al., 2002 and Alonso Diaz de Durana et al., 2003).

(The IgE level to the specific allergen that caused anaphylaxis can "dip" for up to six weeks and therefore a negative skin-prick test or normal IgE level should be delayed or results obtained immediately following a reaction interpreted with more caution than usual.)

'Prick–prick' tests

The 'prick–prick' test involves pricking the fresh food and then pricking the patient's skin with the same lancet (Ives & Hourihane, 2002). The resultant wheal is then examined as with skin-prick tests. It has successfully been used to confirm the suspected allergen following an episode of anaphylaxis (Ewan, 2000a).

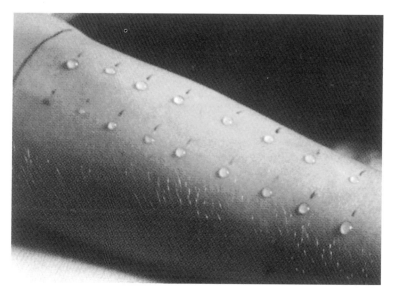

Fig. 8.1 A drop on the allergen solution on the skin of the forearm. Reproduced with permission of Allergy UK

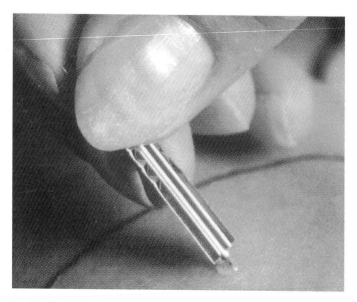

Fig. 8.2 The skin pricked through the allergen solution with a sterile lancet. Reproduced with permission of Allergy UK

Indications for prick–prick tests include:

- Unavailability of skin-prick test for specific commercial extract
- Commercial extract used in a skin-prick test unexpectedly gives a negative result
- When only fresh food is thought to cause a problem (Ives & Hourihane, 2002).

Measurement of serum allergen-specific IgE concentrations

The measurement of serum allergen-specific IgE concentrations has several advantages:

- Not influenced by concurrent drug treatment, i.e. useful when it is not possible to discontinue antihistamine treatment
- Can be performed when the patient has widespread skin disease
- Safe
- High specificity (Rusznak & Davies, 2000 and Kay, 2000).

Pharmacia Cap and DPC ELISA

Pharmacia Cap and DPC ELISA-based testing are the two most widely used methods. The Cap system uses tiny sponges (large surface area) to which the allergen is bound. This is incubated with the patient's serum and then unbound IgE (not directed against the allergen on the sponge) removed by washing. An anti-IgE antibody that has an enzyme attached is then added and binds to any specific IgE that in turn is bound to the sponge. Excess is washed off and the amount of enzyme-labelled antibody bound is proportional to the specific IgE bound. A substrate is added and the enzyme acts on this to produce a colour change, the amount depending on the amount of specific IgE present. The DPC system is based on binding the specific IgE–allergen complexes to an ELISA plate, probably sufficient to say "an ELISA-based method".

Patch tests

Atopy patch tests with food products show promise for enhanced diagnostic accuracy (Sicherer, 2003).

Food challenge

Although a food challenge remains the gold standard for diagnosis of food allergy, it needs very careful consideration in cases of food-induced anaphylaxis (Ives & Hourihane, 2002). However, it is not required if there is a clear history of allergen ingestion and evidence of sensitisation to it (Clark & Ewan, 2002).

Reasons for undertaking a food challenge include:

• Clarifying which foods are causing the reaction
• Identifying which foods may no longer be causing a reaction
• Evaluating non-IgE-mediated reactions where few laboratory tests are available
• Refuting a history of supposed allergy
• Assessing cases where skin tests are positive, but there is no history of ingestion or the history is unclear
• Assessing reactions to other dietary components, e.g. additives, preservatives etc. (Ives & Hourihane, 2002).

Food challenges should be conducted cautiously with incremental doses; adrenaline (epinephrine) and other resuscitation methods should be immediately available.

Measures to avoid exposure to the causative allergen

The cornerstone of treatment for anaphylaxis is the prevention of further attacks by avoiding the allergen. Avoidance is clearly the simplest and most effective strategy for allergy management (Hendry, 2001). Informing family members, friends and work colleagues of the allergen is important.

Minimising the risk of exposure to nuts

Allergy UK have made recommendations in respect of minimising the risk of exposure to nuts:

• Write to the local supermarket requesting a list of products which they consider to be nut-free

- Only buy brands which are either labelled as nut-free on the packaging or are guaranteed as nut-free according to the manufacturer's lists
- If unsure of the contents of a particular product, contact the manufacturer before trying it
- Only eat foods that you are certain about
- Bake your own cakes and biscuits, using a known and safe source of oil or fat, e.g. corn oil, sunflower oil or olive oil
- Inform work colleagues, friends, relatives etc. that you have a nut allergy
- At a restaurant always talk to the chef directly (not the waitress) concerning whether a particular meal is safe; ascertain what type of cooking oil has been used
- Try and use the same restaurants – will help to establish trust with the staff
- If attending a party, take own cake, biscuits etc. if necessary
- In severe peanut allergy, it may be advisable to avoid leguminous foods (Box 8.1).

Minimising the risk of insect stings

The Anaphylaxis Campaign recommends the following to minimise the risk of insect stings:

- Avoid wearing shiny or brightly coloured clothing, flowery prints or black, as this appears to attract bees/wasps more – white, green, tan or khaki clothes are recommended.
- Wear shoes all the time when outdoors.
- Avoid using strong perfumes during the summer months – some suntan lotions, hairsprays and hair tonics can contain strong perfumes.
- If possible keep the arms and legs covered when outdoors.
- Use an insect repellent containing diethyl-m-toluamide if going to be outdoors for a long time (particularly if alone).
- Food attracts wasps/bees – avoid open rubbish bins and keep food covered. Boxed drinks with a straw may be safer than open drink cans. Ensure there are no crumbs or drink on your face.
- The presence of a lot of wasps or bees in the house or garden could indicate that there is a nest nearby, perhaps in the roof or a nearby tree – ask the local authority or pest control expert to remove the nest (source: *Allergy to bee and wasp stings*, a document produced by the Anaphylaxis Campaign with the help of Dr Bill Frankland, Consultant Allergist at Guy's Hospital, London).

Box 8.1   The legume family of foods (peanuts are members of the legume family; those who have a severe peanut allergy may need to avoid other leguminous foods)

Alfafa (sprouts)	Red clover	Tamarind	Cocumarin
Butter beans	Bean sprouts	Tonka bean	Baked beans
Liquorice	Haricot beans	String beans	Chick peas
Black eyed beans	Fenugreek	Jicama	Kuazu
Carob, carob syrup	Gum tragacanth	Lentils	
Gum acacia	Soya beans	Soya bean products	

(Source: *Peanut or nut-free diet*, Allergy UK, 2003b).

Minimising the risk of exposure to latex

Patients with latex allergy need to be aware of common sources of latex (see Fig. 2.2).

In the hospital setting gloves are probably the commonest source of latex. Latex-free gloves are available. In addition, people who are allergic to latex may suffer from cross-reactive allergies to certain foods, including bananas, kiwi fruit and avocados (Allergy UK, 2003a).

Adrenaline (epinephrine) autoinjector devices

An adrenaline (epinephrine) autoinjector device is designed for immediate self-administration by a person with a history of anaphylaxis. It is intended as emergency supportive treatment only, and is not a substitute for medical help (to be sought immediately). Urgent transfer to hospital is essential (Drugs & Therapeutic Bulletin, 2003). The role of adrenaline (epinephrine) autoinjector devices in managing severe anaphylaxis should not be considered in isolation, but rather as a package in which the avoidance of the offending allergen is the priority (Drugs & Therapeutic Bulletin, 2003).

There are currently two autoinjector devices licensed in the UK for self-administration of adrenaline (epinephrine): EpiPen (Alk Abello) and Anapen (Celltech) (Fig. 8.3). The contact details for each company are as follows:

EpiPen	Anapen
Alk Abello (UK) Ltd	Celltech Pharmaceuticals Ltd
2 Tealgate	208 Bath Road
Hungerford	Slough
Berkshire RG17 OYT	Berkshire SL1 3WE
Tel: 01488 686016	Tel: 01753 534655

Both devices are fully assembled syringes that can deliver a single dose of adrenaline (epinephrine) 300 μg IM. Paediatric versions are also available: EpiPen Jr and Anapen Junior, each able to deliver a single dose of 150 μg.

(a)

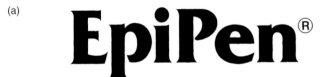

(b)

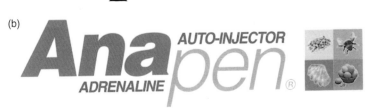

Fig. 8.3   Logos for EpiPen and Anapen (Reproduced by permission of Alk-Abello UK Ltd and Celltech Pharmaceuticals Ltd)

The Project Team of the Resuscitation Council (UK) (2002) suggest:

- The 150 μg device can be administered in children from 6 months to 6 years of age (instead of 120 μg)
- The 300 μg device can be administered in children over 6 years (instead of 250 μg or 500 μg).

Additional fixed-dose self-administration syringes would facilitate more accurate dosing in young children (Simons et al., 2002a).

Provision

In the UK 100 000 adrenaline (epinephrine) autoinjector devices have been prescribed for community use (Unsworth, 2001). These devices have been reported as being both underprescribed (Minhaj & Teuber, 1998) and over-prescribed (Unsworth, 2001). Patient misuse of the devices has also been reported (Huang, 1998).

On reviewing the literature, it is clear that there are controversies concerning the provision of such devices, probably owing to the unavailability of national and international guidelines (Williams, 2002).

According to Sampson's (1992) much-quoted paper, 'epinephrine should be prescribed and kept available for all children and adolescents with IgE-mediated food allergies'. However, because of the large numbers involved, this has huge implications (Williams, 2002).

Potential disadvantages of prescribing adrenaline (epinephrine) for all children with an allergy include:

- More difficult to identify those at high risk of suffering a severe reaction
- Dilution of care available for children at high risk of suffering a severe reaction
- Creation of undue anxiety and limitation of social activities for those with only a mild allergy (Clark & Ewan, 2003).

On reviewing the literature, the following appear to be common indicators for the provision of adrenaline (epinephrine):

- Previous life-threatening event, i.e. laryngeal oedema, respiratory or hypotensive symptoms
- Poorly controlled or severe asthma.

The development of agreed national guidelines regarding the provision of adrenaline (epinephrine) will not only be very helpful for both patients and clinicians, but may also be an important medicolegal issue (Williams, 2002).

In the absence of these guidelines, it would be prudent to follow the advice and recommendations of the local allergist.

How many devices should be prescribed

There appears to be no consensus regarding how many devices should be prescribed. Some advise that a device should be kept at each site that is attended regularly, e.g. workplace, school, home, or with the childminder.

Two devices may be required if the patient is going to a remote region where prompt medical care is not available (Drugs & Therapeutic Bulletin, 2003). Again, following the local allergist's advice is essential.

Training

Training in the use of autoinjector devices is poor (Sicherer et al., 2000, Clegg & Ritchie, 2001 and Clark & Ewan, 2002). In one UK study, only one in eight families was adequately trained (Davies et al., 1996). Trainers themselves must be familiar with the injection devices (Drugs & Therapeutic Bulletin, 2003), though this is not always the case (Sicherer et al., 2000).

It is clearly important to ensure that patients and their relatives/carers (as appropriate) receive adequate training in the use of the autoinjector. Training devices are available from the individual companies. These dummy versions do not have a needle and do not contain the drug.

The patient and carers/relatives should be familiar with how to store the device and be alert to the expiry date (both devices are supplied with a form which can be returned to the companies in order to receive a reminder when the expiratory date of the device is approaching (Drugs & Therapeutic Bulletin, 2003)).

When to use the device

The varied and unpredictable course of severe anaphylaxis makes it difficult to define at what stage the adrenaline (epinephrine) autoinjector should be used (Drugs & Therapeutic Bulletin, 2003). The Project Team of the Resuscitation Council (UK) (2002) recommends that adrenaline (epinephrine) should be administered if there is stridor, respiratory distress, wheeze, or clinical features of shock. Urgent transfer to hospital should also be arranged (Drugs & Therapeutic Bulletin, 2003).

Operating the EpiPen

The EpiPen (Fig. 8.4) is a simple device that is small enough to fit into a pocket or a handbag. A safety cap prevents accidental injection. The procedure for using the EpiPen is as follows:

1. Remove the EpiPen from the packaging
2. Remove the grey safety cap (Fig. 8.5)

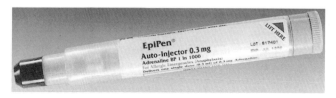

Fig. 8.4   An EpiPen (Reproduced by permission of ALK-Abello UK Ltd)

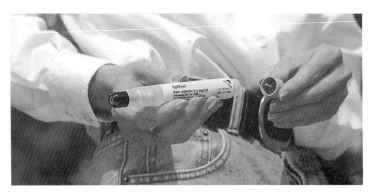

Fig. 8.5 An EpiPen with the safety cap removed (Reproduced by permission of ALK-Abello UK Ltd)

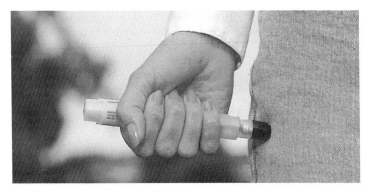

Fig. 8.6 Hold the EpiPen to the thigh until the autoinjector mechanism functions (Reproduced by permission of ALK-Abello UK Ltd)

3. Holding the EpiPen, place the black tip at right-angles to the thigh and press hard until the autoinjector mechanism functions (there should be a click) (Fig. 8.6)
4. Hold the EpiPen in place for 10 seconds
5. Remove the EpiPen and massage the area for 10 seconds
   (Source: Alk Abello product literature).

Although 'fluid' can still be seen in the autoinjector after use, the unit cannot be used again. The EpiPen should be disposed off safely. After use:

1. Gently bend back the needle against a hard surface
2. Carefully insert the device, needle end first (without replacing the safety cap), back into the amber carrying tube
3. Recap the amber carrying tube
4. Dispose of the device at the local hospital when seeking medical help.

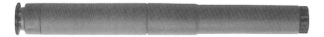

Fig. 8.7   The Anapen

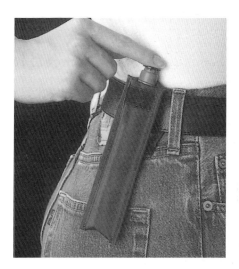

Fig. 8.8   The pouch for carrying the Anapen

Operating the Anapen

The Anapen (Fig. 8.7) has a mechanism whereby, on pushing a button, a spring-activated plunger pushes the needle into the muscle and injects the measured dose of adrenaline (epinephrine) (Drugs & Therapeutics Bulletin, 2003). There are two preparations: Anapen (300 μg) and Anapen Junior (150 μg).

Benefits of the Anapen include:

- Needle cap to maintain sterility
- Simple, one-touch controlled delivery – easy to use and to teach
- Safety cap to prevent accidental 'firing'
- Fine-gauge needle
- Light and compact, with a convenient belt pouch for ease of carrying (Fig. 8.8).

The procedure for using the Anapen is as follows:

1. Remove the black needle cap (Fig. 8.9). This pulls the rubber protective sheath off the needle
2. Remove the black safety cap from the red firing button (Fig. 8.10)
3. Hold the needle end of the device against the outer thigh (Fig. 8.11). If necessary, the injection may be made through light clothing

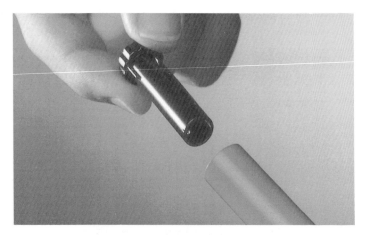

Fig. 8.9 The Anapen with the black needle cap removed

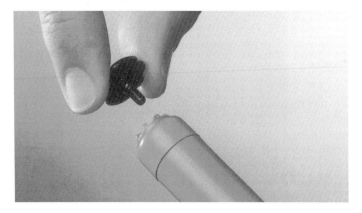

Fig. 8.10 The black safety cap removed from the red firing button

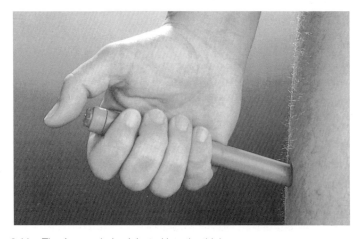

Fig. 8.11 The Anapen being injected into the thigh

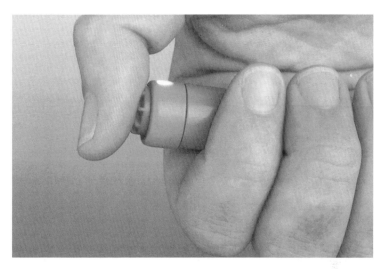

Fig. 8.12 The firing button being pressed down on the Anapen (Figs 8.7–8.12 reproduced with permission from Celltech, Lincoln Medical Ltd)

4. Press the firing button (Fig. 8.12). A spring-activated plunger pushes the needle into the muscle and injects the full dose of adrenaline (epinephrine)
5. Hold the device in position for 10 seconds, then remove it
6. Gently massage the injection site for approximately 10 seconds
7. Replace the black needle cap and discard the device safely immediately after use
   (Source: Celltech Pharmaceuticals product literature).

Principles of desensitisation

Desensitisation or immunotherapy was first described in the first quarter of the last century by researchers at St Mary's Hospital in London (Noon, 1911 and Freeman, 1914). By targeting the allergen that is triggering the reaction, desensitisation provides an alternative to treating the consequences of allergic sensitisation (Frew, 2001). Desensitisation should be considered where possible (Fisher, 1995).

A series of allergen injections are administered to the patient, in which the dose is initially very small and then gradually increased (Parham, 2000). It is usually undertaken over a period of years, usually 3–5 (Howarth, 2000), starting with weekly injections and followed by maintenance injections administered monthly or over longer periods (Ewan, 2000a). Administering the allergen in this way decreases the IgE response over time and causes IgG to be produced instead. It is thought that the IgG binds the allergen and prevents it cross-linking IgE on Mast cells but the exact basis of protection is not clear. TH2 cells stimulate B cells to produce IgE and these cells are inhibited whereas TH1 cells, which favour IgG production are generated.

Box 8.2   Summary of guidelines on specific allergen injection desensitisation

- Use only high-quality standardised allergen extracts
- Only administer in hospitals or specialist clinics
- Ensure adrenaline (epinephrine) is readily available
- Ensure adequate resuscitation services are immediately available (staff attending should be trained in current resuscitation techniques)
- Closely monitor the patient for the first hour following each injection

Cited in Kay A (2000) Good allergy practice. In: Durham S (ed) ABC of Allergies. BMJ Books, London, from Royal College of Physicians and Royal College of Pathologists Good Allergy Practice: Standards of Care Providers and Purchasers of Allergy Services within the National Health Service Royal College of Physicians, London

Unfortunately, because this procedure involves the injection of an allergen to which the patient is already sensitised, there is a risk of anaphylaxis. The procedure can therefore be only undertaken in a controlled environment, where full resuscitation facilities including adrenaline (epinephrine) are available. Box 8.2 summarises the national guidelines on allergen desensitisation.

A more recent approach, which involves vaccination of the patient with allergen-derived peptides, is considered to be safer as it should not trigger anaphylaxis (Parham, 2000).

Desensitisation is the primary treatment for sensitisation to bee and wasp venom (Howarth, 2000), for which it is highly effective (Ewan, 2000a). Venom desensitisation can improve the quality of life for sufferers (Sicherer, 2003). Before it can be undertaken, however, the nature of the sting must be accurately diagnosed and venom-specific IgE demonstrated (Ewan, 2000a). Patients with severe reactions and some with moderately severe reactions will be considered for desensitisation. Other factors to take into account include:

- Risk of future exposure
- Time interval from the last sting
- Other medical problems
- Ability to self-administer treatment
- Access to medical help (Ewan, 2000a).

Desensitisation is not indicated for food allergy (ineffective). Desensitisation to aspirin and NSAIDs is effective in some patients and a few cases of desensitisation to penicillin have been reported.

Key action points to minimise the risk of anaphylaxis

The Anaphylaxis Campaign recommends the following key action points for the patient to minimise the risk of anaphylaxis:

- Take care and be vigilant – avoid the causative agent. The importance of this must be stressed: in an American study of fatal food reactions,

90% of patients (mostly adolescents) had known that they were allergic to the food that killed them (Bock et al., 2001)

- If allergic to food, ask for detailed information from manufacturers and supermarket staff; always read food labels
- Be alert to the initial symptoms; administer adrenaline (epinephrine) without delay if they are serious or becoming serious. Dial 999 or ask someone else to do it
- Ensure other family members know how to administer the adrenaline (epinephrine)
- Ensure colleagues and family members know where the adrenaline (epinephrine) is kept
- Develop a crisis plan on how to handle an emergency – ask the GP or allergist to help. Have this written out for family members, friends and colleagues
- Wear a MedicAlert talisman
- Be open about the problem.

Support organisations

Having suffered a frightening anaphylaxis episode, the possibility of a future one will undoubtedly cause a great deal of anxiety for the patient. Clearly, it is important to reassure patients and stress that they can lead a normal life, with adjustments for allergen avoidance as appropriate. The formulation of an individualised management plan will certainly help to allay fears and concerns. In addition organisations such as the Anaphylaxis Campaign and Allergy UK can be very supportive.

The Anaphylaxis Campaign

The Anaphylaxis Campaign, a registered charity, was set up in 1994 to spread awareness and information about life-threatening allergic reactions. It has two main aims:

- To preserve the health of and relieve those persons who suffer anaphylactic reactions and associated disorders by advancing research into the cause and care of such conditions and to publish the results of such research
- To advance the education and general understanding of the public concerning anaphylaxis and associated disorders.

To achieve these two key aims, the Anaphylaxis Campaign:

- Provides information and guidance via newsletters, fact sheets, leaflets (Fig. 8.13), website and telephone helpline
- Campaigns for better food labelling
- Increases awareness throughout the food and catering industry
- Strives to ensure that those with severe allergies have the best possible advice and treatment
- Promotes research.

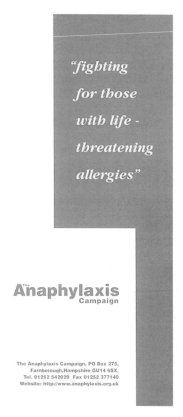

Fig. 8.13   Informative material published by the Anaphylaxis Campaign, with permission

Contact details
The Anaphylaxis Campaign, PO Box 275, Farnborough, Hampshire, GU14 6SX
Tel.: 01252 542029, Fax: 01252 377140
Website: **http://www.anaphylaxis.org.uk**

Allergy UK

Allergy UK, the operational name of the British Allergy Association, is a national medical charity with the principle objectives of:

- Increasing awareness and understanding of allergy
- Helping people manage their allergies
- Raising funds for allergy research
- Providing training in allergy for healthcare personnel, including medical staff, nursing staff, dietitians and pharmacists.

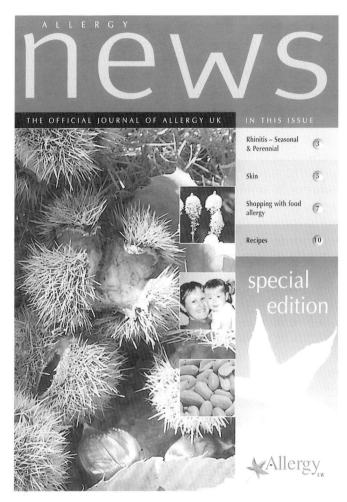

Fig. 8.14   Cover image of Allergy News, with permission of Allergy UK

Benefits from membership of Allergy UK include a fact sheet on the particular allergy, subscription to the regular magazine *Allergy News* (Fig. 8.14) providing information on all aspects of allergies, support contacts throughout the UK and product information. Allergy UK also produces a number of information leaflets (Fig. 8.15).

Contact details
Allergy UK
Deepdene House, 30 Bellegrove Road, Welling, Kent DA16 3PY
Tel.: 020 8303 8525, Helpline tel no: 020 8303 8583
Website: **www.allergyuk.org** Email: **info@allergyuk.org**

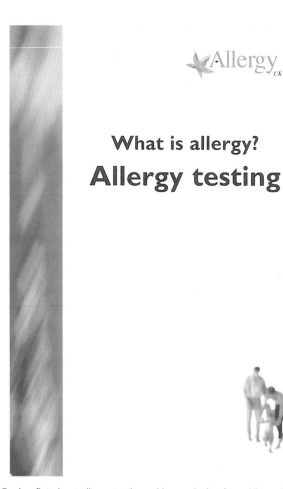

Fig. 8.15   Leaflet about allergy testing, with permission from Allergy UK

MedicAlert

MedicAlert (Fig. 8.16), a registered charity, was founded in 1956 in the USA by Dr M. Collins and Mrs C. Collins after their daughter almost died following an anaphylactic reaction to the horse serum used in a routine tetanus antitoxin test. It currently has a worldwide membership in excess of four million in over 40 countries.

MedicAlert provides a life-saving identification system for individuals with hidden medical conditions and allergies. A MedicAlert member wears a bracelet or necklet (known as an Emblem) (Fig. 8.17), which is engraved with a personal identification number, main medical condition(s) and an emergency telephone number. It also bears the universally recognised symbol of the medical profession.

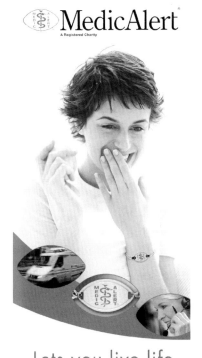

Lets you live life

Fig. 8.16　Leaflet from MedicAlert®, with permission of MedicAlert®

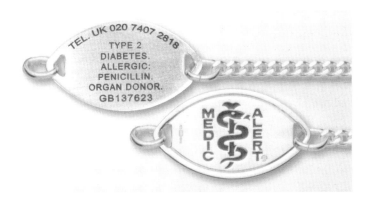

Fig. 8.17　An Emblem used by a MedicAlert® member, with permission of MedicAlert®

In an emergency, medical personnel have immediate access to vital information on the back of the MedicAlert disc. In addition, by telephoning the emergency number (24 hours), they can gain further medical and personal information, e.g. name, address, general practitioner details, current drug therapy and next of kin. A translation service is also available in over 100 different languages.

For further information contact:

MedicAlert, 1 Bridge Wharf, 156 Caledonian Road, London N1 9UU
Tel.: 020 7833 3034
E-mail: **info@medicalert.org.uk** Website: **www.medicalert.org.uk**

Latex Allergy Support Group

The Latex Allergy Support Group (LASG) is a registered charity which aims to:

- Raise awareness of latex allergy among the general public and, in particular, healthcare workers
- Provide a national support network for those affected by latex allergy
- Push for investigation into the increased incidences of the allergy, the identification of 'at risk' groups and the prevention of unnecessary contact with known sensitising agents.

It has produced the following information sheets for latex allergy sufferers:

- *Employment Rights*
- *Health and Safety Legislation*
- *Going into Hospital*
- *Guidance for Schools.*

The Latex Allergy Support Group can be contacted at PO Box 27, Filey Y014 9YH, and on Tel: 07071 225838, Website: **www.lasg.co.uk**

Chapter summary

Patients who have experienced anaphylaxis should be referred to an allergist or clinical immunologist experienced in its management for further investigation and management. The causative agent should be identified and advice given on avoidance to prevent further attacks. Support and education will be required and some patients will need to be equipped with an adrenaline (epinephrine) autoinjector device, together with full instructions in its use.

Chapter 9

Management of anaphylaxis in the school environment

Introduction

The potential for anaphylaxis in the school environment can, understandably, be alarming for children, parents, teachers and other school staff. Parents of children with severe food allergies are often frightened of the dangers their children may encounter in the school environment, and they require support and affirmation (Gaudreau, 2000).

A child who is at risk of anaphylaxis will undoubtedly present a challenge for any school. However, most children with a severe allergy are happily accommodated in mainstream schools thanks to good communication and consensus between parents, teachers, medical staff and education authorities (Anaphylaxis Campaign, 2003).

It is important to ensure that the child can develop in the normal way and is not made to feel different or stigmatised. Effective communication between the education and healthcare services is essential in order to reassure parents and children that, in the event of a reaction, the response will be prompt, efficient and effective (Drugs & Therapeutic Bulletin, 2003). Training programmes will help to achieve this (Vickers et al., 1997).

By the end of this chapter the reader should be able to understand the principles of management of anaphylaxis in the school environment.

Chapter objectives

At the end of the chapter the reader will be able to:

- Discuss how to draw up an individualised management plan
- Outline the support required for school staff
- State the key responsibilities of the school, parents/carers and child
- Outline a sample management plan.

Drawing up an individualised management plan

Many schools have found it essential to draw up an individual management plan or protocol, based on recommendations from the local allergy service, for every child with a severe allergy (Anaphylaxis Campaign, 2003). This is recommended by the Department of Health and Department for Education and Employment (2003). However, not all schools have adopted this approach (Clegg & Ritchie, 2001). Allergy UK and the Anaphylaxis Campaign provide guidance on how to draw up an individualised management plan (Fig. 9.1).

The management plan should address all the important issues, including:

* **Child's details:** name, address, date of birth and brief account of the particular allergy
* **Contact details:** parents'/carers' names and address, telephone numbers (including mobile number), and a second contact name and telephone number

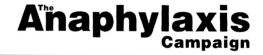

The Anaphylaxis Campaign

Supporting pupils with severe allergies

Anaphylaxis and schools
How we can make it work

Published by
The Anaphylaxis Campaign
PO Box 275
Farnborough, Hants
GU14 6SX

Telephone 01252 542029
Fax 01252 377140
website www.anaphylaxis.org.uk

Fig. 9.1 Guidelines from Allergy UK and the Anaphylaxis Campaign, with permission of the Anaphylaxis Campaign

- **Definition of anaphylaxis:** including signs and symptoms
- **Emergency procedure:** the school must have a clear emergency procedure which all staff must be aware of. It should include assessment of signs and symptoms, recognition of anaphylaxis, administration of any medications as appropriate and the procedure for summoning the emergency services. Hopefully the hospital consultant will have provided the parents/carers with a procedure to follow – this can be incorporated into the management plan
- **Medication:** any medication the child has been prescribed needs to be documented, including when and how to administer it; the medication needs to be clearly labelled with the child's name and instructions for use, and all staff need to know where it is stored. Social services and the employer's insurance company should be informed
- **Food management:** awareness of the child's needs relating to the menu, individual meal requirements and snacks in school; the catering supervisor must be aware of the child's needs. Arrangements for outdoor activities and school trips will need to be planned in advance
- **Staff training:** staff will have training requirements, e.g. recognition of anaphylaxis and use of adrenaline (epinephrine) autoinjector device; the Anaphylaxis Campaign's training video is a useful resource
- **Precautionary measures:** e.g. if the child is allergic to peanuts, it would seem sensible to exclude all peanut products from the school premises to minimise risks; the child could bring in his own food to a party or social event – a supply of 'treats' could be kept for unexpected occasions when birthday cakes or sweets are brought into school
- **Professional indemnity:** required by school staff (see below)
- **Consent and agreement:** the parents/carers must provide written consent for staff to take responsibility for administering medications as required (source: Anaphylaxis Campaign and Allergy UK).

The legal ramifications regarding the child's right for privacy and the right to be educated alongside his peers, as well as laws that protect the non-nursing and non-medical professional who delivers 'medical care', such as using an adrenaline (epinephrine) autoinjector device, need to be explained to the staff (Gaudreau, 2000).

Support required for school staff

School staff have a professional responsibility to safeguard the pupils' health and safety. However, there is no legal obligation that requires school staff to administer medication: it is voluntary (Department of Health and Department for Education and Employment, 2003).

Therefore, teachers who undertake training in the use of medications such as adrenaline (epinephrine) autoinjector devices may wish to seek the support of their professional organisations and employers (Anaphylaxis Campaign, 2003).

The teachers' associations have advised their members who voluntarily undertake this responsibility to:

- Adhere to strictly controlled guidelines
- Seek a professional indemnity from their employers, which will provide legal security in the unlikely event of a claim for alleged negligence (Anaphylaxis Campaign, 2003).

The employer must ensure that their insurance arrangements provide adequate cover for school staff acting within the scope of their employment. Many Local Education Authorities reassure staff working in county and controlled schools who volunteer to assist in the administration of medications that they are acting within the scope of their employment and as such are indemnified (Anaphylaxis Campaign, 2003). An example of a staff indemnity can be found in the sample management plan on pages 97–99.

Responsibilities of the school, parents/carers and the child

The responsibilities relating to the child's allergy should be shared between the school, parents/carers and child (Anaphylaxis Campaign). In their leaflet *Coping with allergies in school* (2003) (Fig. 9.1), the Anaphylaxis Campaign has reviewed these shared responsibilities.

Responsibilities of the school include:

- Ensuring that catering supervisors are aware of an allergic child's dietary requirements
- Reviewing health records submitted by the child's parents/carers
- Ensuring that children with allergies are involved in school activities and not excluded on grounds of their allergy
- Identifying a core team to work closely with parents to establish prevention and treatment strategies
- Ensuring medications are appropriately stored, in a secure location, yet central and easily accessible for designated staff
- Ensuring staff receive adequate training and retraining
- Reviewing the management plan after a reaction occurs.

Responsibilities of the parents/carer include:

- Notifying the school of the details of their child's allergy
- Providing written medical documentation, instructions and medications as directed by the child's doctor
- Educating the child in self-management of the allergy, e.g. what foods are safe and unsafe, how to read food labels, strategies for avoiding allergens, and recognition of the signs and symptoms of a reaction and when to inform an adult
- Working closely with the school to develop a management plan to accommodate the child's specific allergy needs in the classroom, dining room, after-school activities, on the school bus, on school trips etc.

- Replacing medications after use or on expiry
- Providing the school with a supply of some safe snacks for special events, parties etc.

  Responsibilities of the child include:

- Not exchanging food with others
- Avoiding foods with unknown ingredients
- Being proactive in the care and management of their allergy
- Notifying an adult if they inadvertently eat an item of food that could contain the offending allergen
- Notifying an adult if a reaction is starting
- Wearing a MedicAlert bracelet at all times (if they have one).

Sample management plan

The following sample management plan has been reproduced with permission of the Anaphylaxis Campaign.

Case study

This sample protocol was compiled based on working documents now in use for children in Berkshire, Birmingham, Dudley and Hampshire. The schools and Local Education Authorities have kindly shared them with the Anaphylaxis Campaign. It is for guidance only. An individual protocol for each patient must be developed based on the clinical judgement of the patient's GP or consultant.

Background

It is thought probable that John may suffer an anaphylactic reaction if he eats nuts or products containing nuts. If this occurs he is likely to need medical attention and, in an extreme situation, his condition may be life-threatening. However, medical advice is that attention to his diet, in particular the exclusion of nuts, together with the availability of his emergency medication, is all that is necessary. In all other respects, it is recommended by his consultant that his education should carry on 'as normal'.

John also suffers from a mild asthmatic condition and may therefore need occasional access to his inhaler.

The arrangements set out below are intended to assist John, his parents and the school in achieving the least possible disruption to his education, but also to make appropriate provision for his medical requirements.

Details

The head teacher will arrange for the teachers and other staff in the school to be briefed about John's condition and about other arrangements contained in this document.

The school staff will take all reasonable steps to ensure that John does not eat any food items unless they have been prepared/approved by his parents.

John's parents will remind him regularly of the need to refuse any food items that might be offered to him by other pupils.

In particular, John's parents will provide for him a suitable midmorning snack, a suitable packed lunch and suitable sweets to be considered as 'treats', and to be kept by the class teacher.

If there are any proposals which mean that John may leave the school site, prior discussions will be held between the school and John's parents in order to agree appropriate provision and safe handling of his medication.

Whenever the planned curriculum involves cookery or experimentation with food items, prior discussions will be held between the school and parents to agree measures and suitable alternatives.

The school will hold, under secure conditions, appropriate medication, clearly marked for use by designated school staff or qualified personnel and showing an expiry date. A bottle of CLARITYN syrup and two EPIPENS are to be held in the head teacher's office. The parents accept responsibility for maintaining appropriate up-to-date medication.

Allergic reaction

In the event of John showing any physical symptoms for which there is no alternative explanation, his condition will be immediately reported to the head teacher/teacher in charge.

On receipt of such a report, the person in charge, if agreeing that his condition is a cause for concern, will instruct a staff member to contact, in direct order of priority:

Ambulance/Emergency Services 999
GP: 447 5894 / 447 689
Local health centre: 447 889
Message to be given: Anaphylaxis

and then his parents in the following order:

Mother   – 447 665
Father   – 343 675
Grandparents – 656 787

While awaiting medical help the head teacher and designated staff will assess John's condition and administer the appropriate medication in line with perceived symptoms and following closely the instructions given by the paediatrician during the staff training session.

The procedure below will be followed:

- Bad tummy-ache … itchiness … irritated … distressed … tickly throat … vomiting

JOHN WILL BE GIVEN A 5 ML SPOON OF CLARITYN SYRUP

- Wheeziness … pale … drowsy … having difficulty breathing … blue lips … losing consciousness

JOHN WILL BE GIVEN THE EPIPEN ADRENALINE AUTOINJECTION INTO THE OUTER SIDE OF THE THIGH, MIDWAY BETWEEN KNEE AND HIP

The administration of this medication is safe for John, and even if it is given through a misdiagnosis it will do him no harm.

On the arrival of the qualified medical staff the teacher in charge will apprise them of the medication given to John. All medication will be handed to the medical person.

After the incident a debriefing session will take place with all members of staff involved.

Parents will replace any used medication.

Transfer of medical skills

Volunteers from the school staff have undertaken to administer the medication in the unlikely event of John having an allergic reaction.

A training session was attended by seven members of the school staff. Dr T. Fox, the community paediatrician, explained in detail John's condition, the symptoms of the anaphylactic reaction, and the stages and procedures for the administration of medication.

Further advice is available to the school staff at any point in the future where they feel the need for further assistance. The medical training will be repeated at the beginning of the next academic year.

The city council provides a staff indemnity for any school staff who agree to administer medication to a child in school given the full agreement of parents and school.

Staff indemnity

The city council fully indemnifies its staff against claims for alleged negligence, provided they are acting within the scope of their employment, have been provided with adequate training, and are following the LEA's guidelines. For the purposes of indemnity, the administration of medicines falls within this definition and hence the staff can be reassured about the protection their employer provides. The indemnity would cover the consequences that might arise where an incorrect dose is inadvertently given or where the administration is overlooked. In practice indemnity means the city council and not the employee will meet the cost of damages should a claim for alleged negligence be successful. It is very rare for school staff to be sued for negligence, and instead the action will usually be between the parent and the employer.

Agreement and conclusion

A copy of these notes will be held by the school and the parents. A copy will be sent to the local health centre, Dr Fox, the GP, and the Local Education Authority for information.

Any necessary revisions will be the subject of further discussions between the school and the parents.

On a termly basis, any changes in routine will be noted and circulated.

AGREED and SIGNED
On behalf of the school:

Head teacher	date
Chair of the Governors	date
Parents of John Smith	date

Conclusion

A child at risk of anaphylaxis presents a challenge to any school. However, with sound precautionary measures and support from the staff and the doctor responsible, school life may continue as normal for all concerned.

Further information about anaphylaxis and the Anaphylaxis Campaign can be obtained by telephoning the Anaphylaxis Campaign on 01252 542029.

It will be useful to read the above guidance in conjunction with the DfEE/DoH document mentioned above, entitled *Supporting pupils with medical needs in schools*. This is available from DfEE Publications, PO Box 5050, Sherwood Park, Annesley, Notts NG15 0DJ. Tel.: 0845 6022260.

Chapter summary

A child with a severe allergy presents a challenge for any school. An individualised management plan should be drawn up, containing sound precautionary measures and protocols to ensure an effective response in the event of an anaphylactic reaction. The school, parents/carers and child have shared responsibilities to which each must adhere. Hopefully, school life will then continue as normal for all concerned.

Record keeping

Introduction

An accurate written record detailing the management of anaphylaxis, including the later assessment and management, is essential. It forms an integral part of the medical and nursing management of the patient and can help to protect the practitioner if defence of his/her actions is required.

Unfortunately, the exact timing and sequence of events and interventions can sometimes be difficult to recall. Nevertheless, despite this, accurate record keeping will still be expected.

The aim of this chapter is to help the reader understand the principles of good record keeping.

Chapter objectives

At the end of the chapter the reader will be able to:

- Discuss the importance of accurate record keeping
- Outline the principles of effective record keeping
- Detail what post-anaphylaxis records should include
- Discuss the procedure for reporting an adverse reaction to a therapeutic agent
- Discuss when records become a legal document.

Importance of accurate record keeping

Accurate record keeping will help to protect the welfare of the patient by promoting high standards of clinical care and continuity of care through better communication and dissemination of information between members of the multidisciplinary healthcare team. Accurate records will also help the practitioner to detect any changes in the patient's condition promptly. Following an anaphylactic reaction, accurate record keeping can help to determine the most appropriate follow-up and future management of the patient.

Principles of effective record keeping

According to the NMC (2002) (Nursing and Midwifery Council) (Fig. 10.1) there are a number of factors that contribute to effective record keeping. The records should:

- Be factual, consistent and accurate
- Be documented as soon as possible after the event
- Provide current information on the care and condition of the patient
- Be documented clearly and in such a way that the text cannot be erased

OTHER DRUGS (including self-medication & herbal remedies)

Did the patient take any other drugs in the last 3 months prior to the reaction?   Yes/No
If *yes*, please give the following information if known:

Drug (Brand, if known)	Route	Dosage	Date started	Date stopped	Prescribed for

Additional relevant information e.g. medical history, test results, known allergies, rechallenge (if performed), suspected drug interactions. For congenital abnormalities please state all other drugs taken during pregnancy and the date of the last menstrual period.

REPORTER DETAILS
Name and Professional Address: _____

Post code: _____ Tel No: _____
Speciality: _____
Signature: Date:

CLINICIAN (if not the reporter)
Name and Professional Address: _____

Post code: _____
Tel No: Speciality:

If you would like information about other adverse reactions associated with the suspected drug, please tick this box ☐

Send to Medicines Control Agency, CSM FREEPOST, LONDON SW8 5BR or if you are in one of the following NHS regions:
to CSM Mersey, FREEPOST, Liverpool L3 3AB   or CSM Scotland, CARDS, FREEPOST, Edinburg EH3 9YW
or CSM Northern & Yorkshire, FREEPOST 1085, Newcastle upon Tyne NE1 1BR   or CSM Wales, FREEPOST, Cardiff CF4 1ZZ
or CSM West Midlands, FREEPOST SW2991, Birmingham B18 7BR

COMMITTEE ON SAFETY OFMEDICINES   In Confidence   MEDICINES CONTROL AGENCY

SUSPECTED ADVERSE DRUG REACTIONS

If you are suspicious that an adverse reaction may be related to a drug or combination of drugs please complete this Yellow Card. Please report all adverse reactions for black triangle (▼) drugs and only serious adverse reactions for established drugs. For additional reporting advice please see page 10 of the BNF or the MCA website www.open.gov.uk/mca/mcahome.htm. Do not be put off reporting because some details are not known.

PATIENT DETAILS   Patient Initials: _____   Sex: M/F   Weight if known (kg): _____
Age (at time of reaction): _____   Identification (Your Practice / Hospital Ref.)*: _____

SUSPECTED DRUG(S)
Give brand name of drug and batch number if known

	Route	Dosage	Date started	Date stopped	Prescribed for

SUSPECTED REACTION(S)   **Outcome**
Please describe the reaction(s) and any treatment given: Recovered ☐
                                                                  Recovering ☐
                                                                  Continuing ☐
Date reaction(s) started: _____   Date reaction(s) stopped: _____   Other ☐
Do you consider the reaction to be serious?   Yes/No
If *yes*, please indicate why the reaction is considered to be serious (please tick all that apply):

Patient died due to reaction ☐   Involved or prolonged inpatient hospitalisation
Life threatening ☐   Involved persistent or significant disability or incapacity ☐
Congenital abnormality ☐   Medically significant; please give details: ☐

* This is to enable you to identify the patient in any future correspondence concerning this report

Fig. 10.1   Pre-paid yellow card, available from the MCA or BNF

- Have any alterations and additions dated, timed and signed, with all original entries clearly legible
- Be accurately dated, timed and signed (including a printed signature)
- Not include abbreviations, jargon, meaningless phrases or irrelevant speculation.

What post-anaphylactic reaction records should include

It is most important that the anaphylaxis episode is fully documented in the notes. The following should be included:

- Time of reaction, including time help summoned, e.g. emergency services
- Relevant history, including pertinent information related to the possible cause of the reaction. The time from exposure to first symptoms is helpful (if known)
- Presenting clinical features, e.g. bronchospasm, hypotension, laryngospasm, description of any rash
- Details of management, including adrenaline (epinephrine), ECG rhythms and response to treatment
- Any pertinent blood chemistry, e.g. arterial blood gases, pH and base deficit results
- Names of personnel present, including designations
- Details of communication with the patient and relatives
- If applicable, information related to the reporting of an adverse reaction to a therapeutic agent to the Medicines Control Agency.

The clinical records should be legible and accurately reflect what happened during the anaphylaxis episode. In addition, full details of later management and assessment should be included, when appropriate.

Procedure for reporting an adverse reaction to a therapeutic agent

Doctors and pharmacists are urged to report adverse reactions to any therapeutic agent, including:

- Drugs
- Blood products
- Vaccines
- Intrauterine devices
- X-ray contrast media
- Dental or surgical materials
- Herbal products (British Medical Association & Royal Pharmaceutical Society of Great Britain, 2002).

Prepaid yellow cards (Fig. 10.1), available from the Medicines Control Agency (MCA) or from inside the back cover of the *British National Formulary* (BNF), should be completed and forwarded to:

Medicines Control Agency, CSM Freepost, London SW8 5BR.

(The MCA has a 24-hour free phone telephone line (0800 731 6789) available throughout the UK, which offers advice and information on suspected adverse drug reactions.)

Records as a legal document

There is often concern as to what constitutes a legal document. Basically, any document requested by the court becomes a legal document (Dimond, 2003), for example nursing records, medical records, X-rays, laboratory reports – in fact any document that may be relevant to the case. If any of the documents are missing, the writer of the records may be cross-examined as to the circumstances of their disappearance (Dimond, 2003).

'Medical records are not proof of the truth of the facts stated in them but the maker of the records may be called to give evidence as to the truth as to what is contained in them' (Dimond, 2003)

Chapter summary

The importance of good record keeping following an anaphylactic reaction cannot be stressed enough. The record must be:

- Factual
- Legible
- Clear
- Concise
- Accurate
- Signed, timed and dated.

Chapter 11

Legal aspects of anaphylaxis

Bridgit Dimond

Introduction

So many legal issues arise in the area of anaphylaxis that a book could have been written on the law alone. However, in the one chapter permitted, it is my intention to describe very briefly the legal context within which practitioners in this field work, and then take some scenarios of the kinds of legal questions that arise in anaphylaxis and, through these situations, outline the main laws that apply. A list of further reading is provided so that the reader can follow up in more detail topics briefly mentioned here.

Legal system

Laws derive from two main sources: first, Acts of Parliament (known as primary legislation) and regulations (known as secondary legislation) or directions from the European Community, and second the decisions in cases decided by the courts (known as the common law, or judge-made law or case law). The Assemblies of Scotland, Wales and Northern Ireland have varying law-making powers. Primary legislation often gives powers to a minister of the crown to make further more detailed regulations. These are usually drawn up in the form of a statutory instrument, which is laid before Parliament for approval or rejection before it comes into force.

Human Rights Act

This Act came into force on 2 October 2000 (in Scotland on devolution) and has three effects:

- All public authorities or organisations carrying out functions of a public nature are required to respect the European Convention on Human Rights, which is set out in Schedule 1 to the Act.
- Citizens have a right to bring an action in the courts of the UK if they consider that their human rights as set out in the Schedule have been breached by a public authority.
- Judges are required to refer back to Parliament any legislation they consider to be incompatible with the Articles set out in the European Convention on Human Rights.

One of the most significant changes brought about by this Act is that people no longer have to take their case to Strasbourg for a hearing before the European Court of Human Rights, but can avoid the additional cost and delay and bring the case in the UK courts. If a judicial review is sought of a decision that is considered to be in breach of the human rights recognised in the Convention, then legal aid is available for this action.

Of specific significance to anaphylaxis are the following Articles:

- Article 2 – the right to life
- Article 3 – the right not to be subjected to torture or to inhuman or degrading treatment and punishment
- Article 5 – the right to liberty and security of person
- Article 6 – the right to fair and independent hearings
- Article 8 – the right to respect for private and family life and correspondence
- Article 9 – the right to respect for religion, belief etc.
- Article 10 – the right to freedom of expression
- Article 14 – the right not to be discriminated against in the recognition of the Articles.

Box 11.3 illustrates how a patient could use the Articles as the basis of a claim in relation to healthcare services. The articles can be down loaded from the Internet from the Department of Health website, www.doh.gov.uk/humanrights.

Primary care organisation

Under the National Health Service (Primary Care Act 1997), the Health Act 1999, Health and Social Care Act 2001, primary care groups, subsequently given trust status, and care trusts have been established to organise community and primary care services and to commission secondary services. (In Wales local health groups were replaced by Local Health Boards in 2003.) Funds are given to these primary care trusts to arrange for the provision of secondary services for patients in their catchment areas. From April 2002 new strategic health authorities have replaced the commissioning health authorities in England.

GP contracts

General practitioners are mainly self-employed practitioners who have a contract for the provision of services, although increasingly salaried GP posts are being set up.

There is a significant difference between a person being an employee rather than a provider of services. An employee is covered by the vicarious liability of the employer (see below) and therefore would not have to pay personally compensation for harm arising from negligence committed in the course of their employment. In contrast, a self-employed person has to take out his or her own insurance cover. Where the self-employed person is also an employer, then he or she will also be vicariously liable for any negligence of his or her employee(s). Thus a general practitioner who employs practice nurses and receptionists must ensure that he or she has employer's liability insurance cover as well as cover in respect of their own actions. The Medical Defence Union and the Medical Protection Society provide cover for their members.

Accountability – criminal, civil, employer's and professional

When a patient dies or suffers harm as a result of failures by professional staff, then it is likely that various legal proceedings will be held to establish accountability and whether a criminal offence has occurred. Box 11.1 illustrates a situation where there is an investigation following an incident where a patient died as a result of being given an antibiotic to which he

---

Box 11.1   Accountability

Frank, a patient, is given IV penicillin by a nurse. The doctor and the nurse had not checked with the records, where it was clearly documented on the treatment chart that the patient was allergic to penicillin. The patient had informed staff prior to admission. The patient went into anaphylaxis and was admitted to ITU, but died.

was allergic. The situation will be explored to illustrate the criminal, civil, disciplinary and professional proceedings that could take place.

Coroner

In the case of an unexpected death, as in Box 11.1, the death will have to be reported to the coroner. The statutory duty of the coroner is to establish the identity of the deceased and how, where, and when he came by his death; and the particulars, for the time being required by the Registration Acts, to be registered concerning the death. The coroner cannot make a finding that any person is criminally responsible for the death. However, he or she can adjourn the inquest and ask the police and the Crown Prosecution Service to consider criminal proceedings. Changes to the coroner's office are recommended by the 3rd Report of the Shipman Inquiry (Shipman Inquiry Third Report. Death and Cremation Certification. Published 14 July, 2003: www: the-shipman-inquiry.org.uk/reports).

Criminal proceedings

Health professionals can be found guilty of manslaughter if they have acted with such gross negligence in carrying out their professional work that their actions amount to a criminal act. This was the ruling by the House of Lords in the case of R. v Adomako (R. v Adomako [1994] 2 All ER 79), where an anaesthetist was held guilty of manslaughter after a patient had died on the operating table. Clearly, in Frank's case there would appear to have been gross negligence by the doctor who prescribed the antibiotic, and also by the nurse who administered it. They could therefore both face criminal proceedings, where the jury would have to determine whether their conduct was grossly negligent and caused the death of Frank.

Civil proceedings

All health professionals owe a duty of care to their patients. If a patient has suffered harm as a result of negligence by a health professional then the patient could bring an action for negligence against that person or, more usually, the employer of that person. The latter action is possible because of the doctrine of vicarious liability, which makes the employer liable for any harm caused by the negligence of an employee who was acting in the course of his employment. Any claimant would have to show that the employee owed a duty of care, which was broken when the employee failed to follow a reasonable standard of care and caused the reasonably foreseeable harm. To determine whether there has been a breach of the duty of care, the courts have used what has become known as the Bolam test. In the case from which the test takes its name (Bolam v. Friern Hospital Management Committee [1957] 1 WLR 582) Judge McNair said: 'The standard of care expected is the standard of the ordinary skilled man exercising and professing to have that special skill'. If these elements of duty, breach, causation and harm can be established, then compensation is payable to the claimant. In the case of a death, there is a fixed statutory sum payable to the estate of the deceased (at present £10 000), but in addition those persons who were dependent upon the deceased, for example wife and children, can claim in respect of their loss.

Where the harm suffered by the patient is partly the result of their own failings, then if there are failures in the duty of care by a health professional, account would be taken of the patient's own responsibility in causing the harm he or she has suffered. This is known as 'contributory negligence', and the judge would determine the extent to which any compensation payable should be reduced to reflect the patient's fault. In the scenario in Box 11.1 there would appear to be a *prima facie* (at first sight) case of negligence by both the prescribing doctor and the nurse who administered the penicillin. They owed Frank a duty of care; they failed to follow a reasonable standard of care; if this failure caused the death of Frank then negligence would be established and the NHS trust would have to pay out compensation to the family for the harm they caused.

Negligence in communication

Failures in communicating are as much negligence as are failures in practice, as Frank's situation illustrates. It is imperative that every organisation providing health care has a regularly audited system to ensure good communications between staff and patients, and that records are properly kept and regularly referred to by staff. In a recent case a mother notified a nursery that her 5-month old baby was allergic to cow's milk. An assistant gave the baby a cereal that contained milk protein and the baby died. An inquest jury found that the baby died from neglect. The parents have declared their intention of suing the nursery ('Adam Fresco Milk Baby died after nursery's neglect'. *The Times*, 29 January 2003).

Future changes in compensation for clinical negligence

There are currently discussions taking place over whether a statutory scheme for compensation in clinical cases should be introduced which could include no-fault compensation (i.e. it would not have to be established that there was a breach of the duty of care), mediation, compensation calculated according to a tariff, and the payment of structured settlements (Department of Health Press release 2001/0313, 'New Clinical Compensation Scheme for the NHS' 20 July 2001). A further consultation paper recommending an NHS redress scheme was published in 2003 (Department of Health 2003 Making Amends: a consultation paper setting out proposals for reforming the approach to clinical negligence in the NHS. CMO June). At the time of writing further proposals are awaited.

Disciplinary proceedings

The employer of the person whose actions have caused harm would be entitled to take disciplinary action against the employee. There is an implied term in a contract of employment that an employee will act with reasonable care and skill and obey reasonable instructions. An investigation would have to take place, and if it was established that the NHS employee failed to ask the necessary questions or follow the correct procedure, then steps within the disciplinary procedure, from an oral warning to dismissal on the ground of gross misconduct, could take place. A GP who is self-employed does not of course have an employer, but could face disciplinary proceedings brought by the organisation with whom he holds his contract for services. This was previously the health authority, but since Primary Care Trusts (PCT) have been established the contracts will be held by the PCT. Both the nurse and the doctor involved in the case in Box 11.1 would probably face disciplinary proceedings. New contracts of service for GPs are to be introduced in April 2004.

Professional conduct proceedings

Any registered health professional would also face professional conduct proceedings, which could lead to him or her being struck off the register. The actions of the nurse would be reported to the NMC, which has the power to investigate the situation and, if considered appropriate, to hold Conduct and Competence hearings. Similar professional conduct proceedings can be held by the GMC in respect of the doctor concerned.

Expanded role and nurse prescribing

Where health practitioners take on work as an expanded role they must ensure that the same standard of care is provided as would have been available if the person who had originally performed that activity had done it. It is no defence to say to a patient, 'I am sorry that you were harmed, but a staff nurse rather than a doctor undertook that activity and she did not have the training to take the appropriate action in the event of an allergic reaction'. This applies particularly in nurse prescribing, which has seen major changes in recent years.

In the situation in Box 11.2 the prescribing and administering practice nurse is responsible for ensuring that the patient is safe. She should only give the flu injection where it is safe to do so. In addition, she should ensure that the patients have all the information necessary for them to be safe. If the patients fail to wait in the surgery for the requisite time for them to be safe, this may be due to a failure on the nurse's part to warn them of the dangers. Perhaps notices warning about leaving too early, together with leaflets about contraindications for the patient to watch out for, may

---

Box 11.2   Expanded role

A practice nurse prescribes and administers influenza vaccinations. Patients are generally asked to remain in the surgery waiting room for approximately 20 minutes in case of anaphylactic reaction. However, in practice the patients often ignore this advice and leave the surgery immediately after the injection. What is the legal situation if the patient suffers an anaphylactic reaction on the way home?

instil the necessary dangers in the patients' minds. If in spite of receiving all the reasonable notices a patient leaves the surgery too early and suffers an anaphylactic attack on the way home, then it is likely to be seen as the fault of the patient rather than of the nurse.

Another situation where an expanded role may not have been thoroughly thought through is where community nurses are administering injections but are not supplied with anaphylaxis packs. As an anaphylaxis attack could be seen as a reasonably foreseeable possibility, then good practice should ensure that reasonable precautions are taken to reduce the risks of harm, and therefore ensure that community nurses are supplied with the necessary packs and trained in their use.

Nurse prescribing

Initially community nurses and health visitors were given statutory powers to prescribe provided that they had had the necessary additional training. In February 2000 prescribing powers were given to nurses employed by a doctor on the medical list (i.e. GP) and also to nurses working in Walk-in Centres, defined in the regulations as 'A centre at which information and treatment for minor conditions is provided to the public under arrangements made by or on behalf of the Secretary of State'.

As a result of the recommendations of the interim Crown Report (Review of Prescribing, Supply and Administration of Medicines: A Report on the Supply and Administration of Medicines under Group Protocols. Department of Health, London, April 1998) there are now statutory requirements (Prescription-only Medicines (Human Use) Amendment Order 2000 SI 2000 No 1917) for patient group directions under which nurses and other specified health professionals can prescribe. Further information can be obtained from Chapter 28 in Dimond B. *Legal Aspects of Nursing*, 3rd edn, Pearson Education 2001.

The Final Crown Report (Department of Health Review of Prescribing, Supply and Administration of Medicines Final Report (Crown Report) March 1999, Department of Health, London) recommended that there should be statutory changes to enable health professions other than doctors to be identified and trained as independent or dependent prescribers. Legislation to progress these recommendations was contained in Section 63 of the Health and Social Care Act, which amends the Medicines Act 1968.

Further developments in extending prescribing powers came into force on 1 April 2002. A statutory instrument (The Prescription-only Medicines (Human Use) Amendment Order Statutory Instrument 2002 No 549) laid down arrangements for a nurse registered in Parts 1, 3, 5, 8, 10, 11, 12, 13, 14 or 15 of the Professional Register and who is recorded in the Register as qualified to order drugs, medicines and appliances from the *Extended Formulary* to prescribe products listed in the *Extended Formulary*. Schedule 3A of the Statutory Instrument sets out the substances that may be prescribed, administered or directed for administration by *Extended Formulary* nurse prescribers. The Schedule also sets out the conditions for such prescription or administration. The list includes antibiotics, analgesics and vaccines. Full details are published in the *British National Formulary*.

In November 2002 the NMC (Nursing and Midwifery Council, Extended Independent Nurse Prescribing and Supplementary Prescribing. NMC 25/2002, 12 November 2002) issued guidance on standards for the extension of independent prescribing by its registered practitioners. It sets out the standards and content of the programme for extended nurse prescribing and supplementary prescribing, and also the areas, knowledge and competencies required to underpin the practice of prescribing.

It could be argued that as it is reasonably foreseeable that patient could go into anaphylaxis following the administration of a drug by a nurse, then the nurse should be eligible and trained to prescribe and administer life-saving adrenaline (epinephrine). National guidelines are available for the management of anaphylaxis, and failure to follow these could be seen as negligent practice.

A similar problem arises with the use of EpiPens. Many patients who are at risk of anaphylaxis carry an EpiPen for self-administration of adrenaline (epinephrine). However, it could happen that a patient goes into anaphylaxis but is unable to use the EpiPen. A nurse is present but has not had the training to use it. It may be that she knows how to administer the adrenaline (epinephrine) but is not sure that she would be legally authorised to do so. Similar situations could arise in schools, where pupils have EpiPens but teachers do not know how to use them. Questions arise about whether they should all be taught and authorised to assist the pupils.

Department of Health proposals

On 16 April 2002 the Department of Health published proposals to give nurses and pharmacists further prescribing powers to cover some chronic conditions. The proposals were implemented in 2003 and will enable appropriately trained nurses and pharmacists to prescribe for such conditions as asthma, diabetes, high blood pressure and arthritis. Prescriptions for inhalers, hormone replacement therapy and anticoagulants are included in the proposals.

In the situation in Box 11.2 the nurse will have to show that she had the legal powers to prescribe and administer the drug she gave to the patient, that she was following the reasonable standard of care in so doing, that she knew the necessary action to take following an allergic reaction, and that she was not therefore acting illegally or negligently. When a nurse undertakes expanded role activities, she or he must follow the standard that could reasonably have been expected from the health professional who would usually have performed that role.

Multidisciplinary working

Unification of administration is not necessarily a guarantee of cooperation and coordination. Key working and team working depend upon each member of the team appreciating the role that others play in patient care. The law itself does not recognise any rule of team liability: each member of the team is personally and professionally accountable for his or her actions (Wilsher v. Essex Area Health Authority [1986] 3 All ER 801 CA).

Failures in communication can often lead to harm to the patient, and the Health Service Commissioners reports show that poor communications are often one of the main reasons why complaints arise.

Patients' rights

Right to services/drugs/operations (Box 11.3)

The Secretary of State has a statutory duty under NHS legislation to provide a comprehensive National Health Service to meet all reasonable requirements, which covers both prevention and treatment and specifically requires a number of services to be provided. However, there have been a series of cases where the courts have held that, provided the Secretary of State has fulfilled his/her statutory duty to provide a comprehensive National Health Service to meet all reasonable requirements, and provided there is no obvious evidence of irrational or unreasonable setting of priorities, then the courts will not be involved in the determination of the allocation of resources.

Thus in the inevitable situation where resources are finite and demand outmatches supply, providers and commissioners of services have to weigh priorities. Examples of when individual patients have sought to enforce the statutory duty to provide services, and the courts have refused to intervene, include a case where patients sued the Secretary of State and other health organisations because they had waited too long for hip operations. They failed in their claim (R. v. Secretary of State for Social Services *ex parte* Hincks and others. 29 June 1979 (1979) 123 *Solicitors Journal* 436).

In another case, a Mrs Walker failed to obtain a declaration that heart surgery should be carried out on her child (R. v. Central Birmingham Health Authority *ex parte* Walker (1987) 3 BMLR 32; *The Times* 26 November 1987).

More recently, Jamie Bowen, a child suffering from leukaemia, was refused by the purchasers a course of chemotherapy and a second bone marrow transplant on the grounds that there was only a very small chance

---

Box 11.3 A right to services

Ben Brown suffered from an allergy to nuts. He had learnt that, following research in the United States, it was possible to take a daily pill which would have the effect of suppressing the allergy, so that he did not need to worry what he ate. He discovered that the medicine was available in the UK and asked his doctor to prescribe it. The doctor said that it cost over £4,000 a year and the Primary Care Trust would not allocate resources for it to be prescribed. It was cheaper and healthier for Ben to stay on the diet. Ben is prepared to challenge this refusal to prescribe.

of the treatment succeeding, and therefore it would not be in her best interests for the treatment to proceed. The Court of Appeal upheld the decision of the Health Authority (R. v. Cambridge HA *ex parte* B [1995] 2 All ER 129).

Cases succeeding on grounds of failure to provide services

More recently, however, there have been several cases where the courts have upheld the right of an individual patient to access services. The first was in relation to the failure of a Health Authority to permit a drug for multiple sclerosis to be prescribed in its catchment area (R. v. North Derbyshire Health Authority [1997] 8 Med L R 327). The Health Authority decided that it would not allow β-interferon to be prescribed for patients in its catchment area, as it was not yet proved to be clinically effective for the treatment of multiple sclerosis. A patient with multiple sclerosis challenged this refusal and succeeded on the grounds that the Health Authority had failed to follow the guidance issued by the Department of Health (NHS Executive Letter: EL (95)97).

In the second case a Health Authority refused to fund treatment for three transsexuals who wished to undergo gender reassignment (North West Lancashire Health Authority v. A, D, and G [1999] Lloyds Law Reports Medical page 399). The transsexuals sought judicial review of the Health Authority's refusal and the judge granted an order quashing the Authority's decision and the policy on which it was based. The Health Authority then took the case to the Court of Appeal, but lost. The Court of Appeal held that although the precise allocation and weighting of priorities is a matter for the judgement of the Authority and not for the court, it is vital for an Authority:

- To assess accurately the nature and seriousness of each type of illness
- To determine the effectiveness of various forms of treatment for it
- To give proper effect to that assessment and that determination in the formulation and individual application of its policy.

The Authority's failure to treat transsexualism as an illness, and its policy, amounted to a 'blanket policy' against funding treatment for the condition because it did not believe in such treatment. There was no evidence that it genuinely considered individual exceptions. The court, however, held in respect of the Human Rights arguments that Articles 3 and 8 of the European Convention on Human Rights did not give a right to free health care and did not apply to this situation, where the challenge is to a Health Authority's allocation of finite funds. Nor were the patients victims of discrimination on the grounds of sex.

Returning to the scenario in Box 11.3, Ben would have to show that the Primary Care Trust and his doctor failed to consider his individual circumstances when they refused to allow him to have the new medication, and that there had been a failing in terms of following the appropriate policy. Clearly he would be helped if there were NICE (National Institute for Clinical Excellence) recommendations stating that there were clear advantages for allergic patients to be prescribed the new medication, which was effective. In the absence of such guidelines he is unlikely to succeed. The High Court has recently held that patients who wait an unreasonable length of time for NHS treatment are entitled to go abroad to an EC country and be refunded by the NHS (R (Watts) v. Bedford Primary Care Trust. The Times Law Report 30 October 2003).

Consent: living wills; autonomy; mentally incapacitated adult

It is a basic principle of the common law that a mentally competent adult has the right to give or refuse consent to treatment. Even if the mentally competent adult requires life-saving treatment, that person has the right to refuse: the only requirement is that there should be clear evidence of mental competence. Thus where a tetraplegic patient was dependent upon a ventilator she was entitled to ask for it to be switched off (In re B (Consent to treatment: Capacity) [2000] 2 All ER 449). Two psychiatrists confirmed that she had the requisite mental capacity. The following tests of mental capacity were used by the Court of Appeal in a case where a pregnant woman refused to have a caesarean section because she suffered a needle phobia (Re MB (an adult: medical treatment) [1997] 2 FLR 426) and (Re MB (an adult: medical treatment) (1997) 38 BMLR 175 CA):

A person lacks the capacity if some impairment or disturbance of mental functioning renders that person unable to make a decision whether to consent to or to refuse treatment. That inability to make a decision will occur when:

1. The patient is unable to comprehend and retain the information that is material to the decision, especially as to the likely consequences of having or not having the treatment in question.
2. The patient is unable to use the information and weigh it in the balance as part of the process of arriving at the decision.

Mental incapacity

Where a person lacks the mental capacity to make a decision, then action must be taken in his or her best interests (Re F (mental patient: sterilisation) [1990] 2 AC 1). There have been proposals for legislation to provide a statutory framework for decision making on behalf of mentally incapacitated adults (Lord Chancellor's Office. *Making Decisions: The Government's Proposals for Decision Making on Behalf of the Mentally Incapacitated Adult.* October 1999, Stationery Office, London). In Scotland an Adults with Incapacity (Scotland) Act 2000 has come into force, but the rest of the UK still has to rely upon common law powers to act in the best interests of a mentally incapacitated adult.

Box 11.4   Refusing a transplant (Re M (medical treatment: consent) [1999] 2 FLR 1097)

A girl of 15 refused to consent to a transplant which was needed to save her life. She stated that she did not wish to have anyone else's heart and she did not wish to take medication for the rest of her life. The hospital, which had obtained her mother's consent to the transplant, sought leave from the court to carry out the transplant.

The court held that the hospital could give treatment according to the doctor's clinical judgement, including a heart transplant. The girl was an intelligent person whose wishes carried considerable weight, but she had been overwhelmed by her circumstances and the decision she was being asked to make. Her severe condition had developed only recently and she had had only a few days to consider her situation. While recognising the risk that for the rest of her life she would harbour resentment about what had been done to her, the court weighed that risk against the certainty of death if the order were not made.

Children

Young persons of 16 and 17 have a statutory right under the Family Law Reform Act 1969 to give consent to treatment. Treatment is widely defined and covers surgical, medical and dental treatment, anaesthesia and diagnostic procedures. Where a young person gives consent, then there is no requirement for the parents also to consent. Where the young person is unable to give consent, then parents can consent on the child's behalf until the child is an adult at 18 years.

Although young persons and children under 16 do not have a statutory right to give consent, they do have a right recognised at common law by the House of Lords in the Gillick case (Gillick v. W. Norfolk and Wisbech Area Health Authority [1986] 1 AC 112), provided that they have the mental capacity to understand the information and the risks involved, i.e. that they are 'Gillick competent'. For 16- and 17-year-olds there is a presumption of capacity which can be rebutted; for the child under 16 the requisite mental capacity must be established.

Child refusing transplant

Although a young person of 16 or 17 has a statutory right to give consent, and a child of any age has a right recognised at common law to give consent if Gillick competent, the principle has been set by the Court of Appeal that if life-saving treatment is necessary and in the best interests of the child, then a person under 18 years cannot give a valid refusal. Thus treatment was forced upon an anorexic girl of 16 years. In the case shown in Box 11.4 a young girl of 15 was compelled to have a heart transplant against her will.

Confidentiality

All health professionals are bound by a duty of confidentiality in relation to information learnt about the patient and given them in confidence.

Box 11.5   Confidentiality

Mohammed had an anaphylactic attack and is being treated in hospital. Although still not fully recovered, he wishes to take his own discharge from hospital because he wishes to return to his job as a taxi driver. He has been advised by his doctor that he should not drive home. However, the doctor knows that he is likely to ignore this advice.

This duty derives from many sources:

• Trust relationship between patient and professional
• Implied term in the contract of employment
• Statutory provisions such as the Data Protection Act 1998
• Professional codes of conduct
• Duty of care to the patient may include a recognition that the duty of care includes the safekeeping of confidential information.

The law recognises many exceptions to this duty, which are:

• The consent of the patient
• Disclosure in the interests of the patient, e.g. to the multidisciplinary team
• The requirement of the court for information to be given
• Several Acts of Parliament recognise a situation where confidential information can be passed on, for example informing the police about a road accident in which there has been personal injury; information passed under the Prevention of Terrorism legislation; notification of infectious diseases under public health legislation
• Disclosure in the public interest, e.g. reporting concerns about child protection; or where serious harm to the physical or mental health of the patient or another person is feared.

In the situation in Box 11.5 there is a clear danger to public safety if Mohammed continued to drive, and the doctor should be protected under the need to protect the safety of the public if he were to report Mohammed to the Driving and Vehicle Licensing Authority. The doctor should of course first attempt to persuade Mohammed to stay in hospital and not to drive, warning him that he commits a criminal offence if he drives when advised that he is medically unfit to do so, and alerting him to the fact that the doctor himself could report it if Mohammed himself failed to stop driving until he was medically fit.

Complaints

At the time of writing a new complaints scheme for the NHS is being drafted (Department of Health. *Reforming the NHS Complaints Procedure: a listening document*. Department of Health, London, September 2001). It follows research over several years on the scheme established in 1996 following the Wilson Report into complaints (Department of Health. *Being Heard. The report of a review committee on NHS Complaints procedures.* May 1994, Department of Health, London). It is likely to involve the Primary Care Trust (in Wales the Local Health Board from 1 April 2003) in being responsible for the initial investigation and then ensuring that independence is an essential feature for further review. The Department of Health has subsequently published its proposals for reform (DoH 2003 NHS Complaints Reform – Making Things Right. DoH).

Health and safety

All health professionals in primary care are subject to health and safety legislation. The main duties placed on both employer and employee are set out in the Health and Safety at Work Act 1974. These statutory duties are supplemented by regulations. These include the Manual Handling Regulations, in which guidance is provided by the Health and Safety Executive (Health and Safety Executive. *Manual Handling: Guidance on Regulations.* HMSO, London, 1992). In addition to the statutory duties there are implied terms in the contract of employment that an employer will take reasonable care of the health and safety of employees. In the situation in Box 11.6, clearly social services or the agency providing the care assistants have a statutory duty and also a contractual duty to ensure that reasonable care is taken of the health and safety of employees, and therefore that, where manual handling can be reasonably avoided, that is done and that other steps are taken to reduce the risk of harm from any remaining manual handling. It would appear a reasonable request to use a hoist. It is unlikely that Mary and her father would succeed in arguing that they had a right under the European Convention of Human Rights for a hoist not to be used, as with skilful use hoisting should not be seen as degrading or inhumane treatment under Article 3.

Manual handling is only one of many areas of health and safety laws relevant to health care, and each trust and PCT should ensure that there is an identified officer who ensures compliance with risk assessment and management principles, the medical devices regulations, the reporting of incidents, injuries and diseases and other legislation. The National Patient Safety Agency will require reports of incidents and hazards to be notified, so that they can ensure that such incidents do not occur elsewhere.

Box 11.6 A lifting nightmare

Mary cares for her elderly father who is severely disabled with multiple sclerosis. She has support from social services three times a day. She has been informed that they want a hoist to be installed and will not allow their care staff to handle her father manually. Both she and her father object to the use of the hoist, and Mary says that she has never had difficulties in raising and lifting him on her own. Her father says that it is contrary to his human rights to be forced to be hoisted.

Conclusions

This chapter is but a superficial description of some of the laws that are relevant to those involved in anaphylaxis, but it is hoped that it will provide a path through the legal maze to more detailed knowledge.

Further reading

Dimond B (2001) Legal Aspects of Nursing, 3rd edn. Pearson Education, London

Dimond B (2002) Legal Aspects of Patient Confidentiality. Quay Publications, Mark Allen Press, Dinton, Salisbury

Dimond B (2002) Legal Aspects of Pain Management. Quay Publications, Mark Allen Press, Dinton, Salisbury

Dimond B (2003) Legal Aspects of Consent. Quay Publications, Mark Allen Press, Dinton, Salisbury

Health and Safety Commission (1992) Manual Handling Regulations and approved code of practice. HMSO, London

Hurwitz B (1998) Clinical Guidelines and the Law. Radcliffe Medical Press, Oxford

Kennedy I, Grubb A (2000) Medical Law and Ethics, 3rd edn. Butterworths, London

McHale J, Tingle J (2001) Law and Nursing. Butterworth–Heinemann, Oxford

Pitt G (2000) Employment Law, 4th edn. Sweet and Maxwell, London

Selwyn N (2000) Selwyn's Law of Employment, 11th edn. Butterworths, London

Wilkinson R, Caulfield H (2000) The Human Rights Act: a Practical Guide for Nurses. Whurr Publishers, London

References

Adams B (2002) Exercise-induced anaphylaxis in a marathon runner. Int J Dermatol 41: 394–6

Advanced Life Support Group (ALSG) (2001) Advanced Paediatric Life Support: A Practical Approach, 3rd edn. BMJ Books, London

Agostini A, Cicardi M (1992) Hereditary and acquired C-1 inhibitor deficiency: biological and clinical characteristics in 235 patients. Medicine 71: 206–15

AHA & ILCOR (American Heart Association & International Liaison Committee on Resuscitation) (2000) Guidelines 2000 for Cardiopulmonary Resuscitation and Emergency Cardiovascular Care – an international consensus on science. Resuscitation 46: 1–448

Allergy UK (2003a) What is Allergy? Allergy UK, Kent

Allergy UK (2003b) Latex Allergy Newsletter. Allergy UK, Kent

Allergy UK (2003c) Peanut or Nut Free Diet. Allergy UK, Kent

Alonso Diaz de Durana M, Fernandez-Rivas M, Casas M et al. (2003) Anaphylaxis during negative penicillin skin prick testing confirmed by elevated serum tryptase. Allergy 58: 159

Alves B, Sheikh A (2001) Age specific aetiology of anaphylaxis. Arch Dis Child 85: 348

American Academy of Pediatrics (1997) Pediatric Advanced Life Support. American Heart Association, USA

American College of Surgeons (1997) Advanced Trauma Life Support. American College of Surgeons, USA

Anaphylaxis Campaign (2003) Anaphylaxis and Schools, How We Can Make it Work. Anaphylaxis Campaign, Farnborough

Antevil J, Muldoon M, Battaglia M, Green R (2003) Intra-operative anaphylactic shock associated with bacitracin irrigation during revision total knee arthroplasty. A case report. J Bone Joint Surg [Am] 85-A: 339–42

Association of Anaesthetists of Great Britain and Ireland and British Society of Allergy and Clinical Immunology (1995) Suspected Anaphylactic Reactions Associated with Anaesthesia. Association of Anaesthetists of Great Britain and Ireland, London

Atkinson T, Kaliner M (1992) Anaphylaxis. Med Clin North Am 76: 841

Bacal E, Patterson R, Zeiss C (1978) Evaluation of severe (anaphylactic) reactions. Clin Allergy 8: 295

Barach E, Nowak R, Lee T et al. (1984) Epinephrine for treatment of anaphylactic shock. JAMA 251: 2118–22

Barnadas M, Cistero A, Sitjas D et al. (1995) Systemic capillary leak syndrome. J Am Acad Dermatol 32: 364–6

Beck S, Burks A (1999) Taking action against anaphylaxis. Contemp Pediatr 16: 87

Bernardini R, Novembre E, Lombardi E et al. (2002) Anaphylaxis to latex after ingestion of a cream-filled doughnut contaminated with latex [letter]. J Allergy Clin Immunol 110: 534–5

Bird A (1996) Anaphylaxis. In: Skinner D, Swain A, Robertson C, Peyton R (Eds) Cambridge Textbook of Accident & Emergency Medicine. Cambridge University Press, Cambridge

Board of Faculty of Clinical Radiology, Royal College of Radiologists (1996) Advice on the Management of Reactions to Intravenous Contrast Media. Royal College of Radiologists, London

Bochner B, Lichtenstein L (1991) Anaphylaxis. N Engl J Med 324: 1785–90

Bock S, Sampson H, Atkins F et al. (1988) Double-blinded, placebo-controlled food challenge (DBPCFC) as an office procedure: a manual. J Allergy Clin Immunol 82: 987–97

Bock S, Munoz-Furlong A, Sampson H (2001) Fatalities due to anaphylactic reactions to foods. J Allergy Clin Immunol 107: 191–3

Brazil E, MacNamara A (1998) 'Not so immediate' hypersensitivity – the danger of biphasic anaphylactic reactions. J Accident Emerg Med 15: 252–3

Briner W (1995) Physical allergies and exercise: clinical implications for those engaged in sports activities. Sports Med 15: 365–73

British Medical Association & Royal Pharmaceutical Society of Great Britain (2001) British National Formulary. British Medical Association, London

British Medical Association & Royal Pharmaceutical Society of Great Britain (2002) British National Formulary. British Medical Association, London

Brown A (1998) Therapeutic controversies in the management of acute anaphylaxis. J Accident Emerg Med 15: 89–95

Bush W, Swanson D (1991) Acute reactions to intravascular contrast media: types, risk factors, recognition and specific treatment. Am J Roentgenol 157:1153–61

Casale T, Keahey T, Kaliner M (1986) Exercise-induced anaphylactic syndromes. JAMA 255: 2049–53

Castells M, Horan R, Sheffer A (2003) Exercise-induced anaphylaxis. Curr Allergy Asthma Rep 3: 15–21

Chamberlain D (2001) Anaphylaxis management in primary care. Prof Nurse 16: 1214–15

Clark A, Ewan P (2002) The prevention and management of anaphylaxis in children. Current Paediatrics 12: 370–5

Clark A, Ewan P (2003) Food allergy in childhood. Have the dangers been underestimated? Arch Dis Child 88: 79–80

Clark A, Nasser S (2001) Anaphylaxis. The State of Allergy/Immunotherapy in the UK. Rila Publications Ltd, London

Clegg S, Ritchie J (2001) 'EpiPen' training; a survey of the provision for parents and teachers in West Lothian. Ambulatory Child Health 7: 169–75

Cogen F, Beezhold D (2002) Hair glue anaphylaxis: a hidden latex allergy. Ann Allergy, Asthma Immunol 88: 61–3

Colquhoun M, Jevon P (2000) Resuscitation in Primary Care. Butterworth Heinemann, Oxford

Cox C, Grady K (2002) Managing Obstetric Emergencies, 2nd edn. BIOS Scientific Publishers, London

Cregler L (1991) Cocaine: the newest risk factor for cardiovascular disease. Clin Cardiol 14: 449–56

Davies R (1999) The British Medical Association Family Doctor Guide to Allergies and Hay Fever. Dorling Kindersley, London

Davies H, Harris J, Kakoo A (1996) Patients should be taught how to inject adrenaline. Br Med J 312: 638

Department of Health (1996) Immunisation against infectious disease. HMSO, London

Department of Health and Department for Education and Employment (2003) A good practice guide. Supporting pupils with medical needs (online). Available http://www.dfee.gov.uk/medical/med.pdf (accessed 28 May 2003)

Dimond B (2003) Legal Aspects of Midwifery, 3rd edn. Butterworth Heinemann, Oxford

Ditto A (2002) Hymenoptera sensitivity: diagnosis and treatment. Allergy Asthma Proc 23: 381–4

Douglas D, Sukenick E, Andrade W et al. (1994) Biphasic systemic anaphylaxis: an inpatient and outpatient study. J Allergy Clin Immunol 93: 977–85

Drugs & Therapeutic Bulletin (1994) 32: 19–21

Drugs & Therapeutic Bulletin (2003) 41: 21–24

Durham S (ed) (2000) ABC of Allergies. BMJ Books, London

Dutau G, Michaeu P, Juchet A et al. (2001) Exercise and food-induced anaphylaxis. Pediatr Pulmonol (Suppl 23): 48–51

Edwards K, Johnston C (1997) Allergic and immunologic disorders. In: Barkin R (ed) Pediatric Emergency Medicine, 2nd edn. Mosby, London

Emerman C, Bellon E, Lukens T et al. (1990) The effect of bolus injection on circulation times during cardiac arrest. Am J Emerg Med 8: 190–3

European Resuscitation Council (2001) Guidelines 2000 for Adult and Paediatric Basic Life Support and Advanced Life Support. Resuscitation 48: 199–239

Ewan PW (1996) Clinical study of peanut and nut allergy in 62 consecutive patients; new features and associations. Br Med J 312: 1074–8

Ewan P (2000a) Anaphylaxis. In: Durham S (ed) ABC of Allergies. BMJ Books, London

Ewan P (2000b) Venom allergy. In: Durham S (ed) ABC of Allergies. BMJ Books, London

Ewan P, Clark A (2001) Long-term prospective observational study of patients with peanut and nut allergy after participation in a management plan. Lancet 357: 111–15

Fiocchi A, Bouygue G, Restani P et al. (2003) Anaphylaxis to rice by inhalation. J Allergy Clin Immunol 111: 193–5

Fiocchi A, Restani P, Ballabio C et al. (2001) Severe anaphylaxis induced by latex as a contaminant of plastic balls in play pits. J Allergy Clin Immunol 108: 298–300

Fisher M (1986) Clinical observations on the pathophysiology and treatment of anaphylactic cardiovascular collapse. Anaesth Intens Care 14: 17–21

Fisher M (1995) Treatment of acute anaphylaxis. Br Med J 311: 731–3

Fisher M (1997) Anaphylaxis. In: Oh T (ed) Intensive Care Manual, 4th edn. Butterworth Heinemann, Oxford

Fisher M, Baldo B (1993) The diagnosis of fatal anaphylactic reactions during anaesthesia: employment of immunoassays for mast cell tryptase and drug-reactive IgE antibodies. Anaesth Intens Care 21: 353–7

Freeman J (1914) Vaccination against hay fever: report of results during the first three years. Lancet 1: 1178

Freishtat R, Goepp J (2002) Episodic stridor with latex nipple use in a 2 month old infant. Ann Emerg Med 39: 441–3

Frew A (2001) The need for allergen immunotherapy in the UK. The state of allergy/immunotherapy in the UK. Rila Publications, London

Garvey L, Roed-Peteren J, Husum B (2001) Anaphylactic reactions in anaesthetised patients – four cases of chlorhexidine allergy. Acta Anaesth Scand 45: 1290–4

Gaudreau J (2000) The challenge of making the school environment safe for children with food allergies. J School Nurs 16: 5–10

Gellert G, Rall J, Brown C et al. (1992) Scombroid fish poisoning: underreporting and prevention among non-commercial and recreational fishers. West J Med 157: 645–7

Grundy J, Bateman B, Gant C et al. (2001) Peanut allergy in three-year-old children – a population based study. J Allergy Clin Immunol 107: S231

Gu X, Simons K, Simons F (2002) Is epinephrine administration by sublingual tablets feasible for the first-aid treatment of anaphylaxis? A proof-of-concept study. Biopharmaceutics & Drug Disposition 23: 213–16

Gupta R, Sheikh A, Strachan D, Anderson H (2003) Increasing hospital admissions for systemic allergic disorders in England: analysis of national admissions data. Br Med J 327: 1142–3

Henderson N (1998) Anaphylaxis. Nurs Standard 12: 49–55

Hendrix S, Sale S, Zeiss C, Utley J, Patterson R (1981) Factitious Hymeroptera allergic emergency: a report of a new variant of Munchausen's Syndrome. Allergy Clin Immunol 67(1): 8–13

Hendry C (2001) Understanding allergies and their treatment. Nurs Standard 15: 47–54

Hendry C, Farley A (2001) Understanding allergies and their treatment. Nurs Standard 15(35): 47–54

Hepner M, Ownby D, Anderson J et al. (1990) Risk of systemic reactions in patients taking beta-blocker drugs receiving allergen immunotherapy injections. J Allergy Clin Immunol 86: 407–11

Holgate S (2001) Improving Clinical Allergy Services for Patients in the UK. The State of Allergy/Immunotherapy in UK. Rila Publications, London

Hong S, Wong J, Bloch K (2002) Reactions to radiocontrast media. Allergy Asthma Proc 23: 347–51

Horan R, Pennoyer D, Sheffer A (1991) Management of anaphylaxis. Immunol Allergy Clin North Am 2: 117–41

Hough D, Dec K (1994) Exercise-induced asthma and anaphylaxis. Sports Med 18: 162–72

Hourihane J, Dean T, Warner J (1996) Peanut allergy in relation to heredity, maternal diet and other atopic diseases: results of a questionnaire survey, skin prick testing and food challenges. Br Med J 313: 6–9

Howarth P (2000) Pathogenic mechanisms: a rational base for treatment. In: Durham S (ed) ABC of Allergies. BMJ Books, London

Howarth P, Evans R (1994) Key Topics in Accident & Emergency Medicine. BIOS Scientific, Oxford

Howatson-Jones I (2000) Adverse reactions to contrast media. Prof Nurse 15: 771–4

Huang S (1998) A survey of EpiPen use in patients with a history of anaphylaxis. J Allergy Clin Immunol 102: 525–6

Hunt L (1993) The epidemiology of latex allergy in healthcare workers [Editorial]. Arch Pathol Lab Med 117: 874–5

Ii M, Sayama K, Tohyama M, Hashimoto K (2002) A case of cold-dependent exercise-induced anaphylaxis. Br J Dermatol 147: 368–70

Ives A, Hourihane J (2002) Evidence-based diagnosis of food allergy. Curr Paediatr 12: 357–64

James J, Zeiger R, Lester M et al. (1998) Safe administration of influenza vaccine to patients with egg allergy. J Pediatr 133: 624–8

Jarvis D, Burney P (2000) The epidemiology of allergic disease. In: Durham S (ed) ABC of Allergies. BMJ Books, London

Jevon P (2002) Advanced Cardiac Life Support. Butterworth Heinemann, Oxford

Jevon P (2003) Paediatric Advanced Life Support. Butterworth Heinemann, Oxford

Jevon P, Ewens B (2002) Monitoring the Critically Ill Patient. Blackwell Publishing, Oxford

Jevon P, Ewens B, Manzie J (2000) Peak flow. Nurs Times 96: 49–50

Johnston S, Unsworth J, Gompels M (2003) Adrenaline given outside the context of life-threatening allergic reactions. Br Med J 326: 589–90

Joint Taskforce on Practice Parameters, American Academy of Allergy, Asthma and Immunology and the Joint Council of Allergy, Asthma and Immunology (1998) The diagnosis and management of anaphylaxis. J Allergy Clin Immunol 101: S465

Jones G (2002) Anaphylactic shock. Emerg Nurse 9: 29–35

Katayama H, Yamaguchi K, Kozuka T et al. (1990) Adverse reactions to ionic and non-ionic contrast media. A report from the Japanese Committee on the Safety of Contrast Media. Radiology 175: 621–8

Kay A (2000) Good allergy practice. In: Durham S (ed) ABC of Allergies. BMJ Books, London

Kelly K, Pearson M, Kurup P et al. (1994) A cluster of anaphylactic reactions in children with spina bifida during general anaesthesia: epidemiological features, risk factors and latex hypersensitivity. J Allergy Clin Immunol 94: 53–61

Kelso J (1999) The gelatin story. J Allergy Clin Immunol 103: 200–2

Kemp S, Lockey R, Wolf B et al. (1995) Anaphylaxis: a review of 266 cases. Arch Intern Med 155: 1749–54

Khakoo G, Lack G (2000) Recommendations for using MMR vaccine in children allergic to eggs. Br Med J 320: 929–32

Khun G, White B, Swetman R (1981) Peripheral vs central circulation times during CPR: a pilot study. Ann Emerg Med 10: 417–19

Lalli A (1980) Contrast media reactions: data analysis and hypothesis. Radiology 134: 1–12

Lamson R (1924) Sudden death associated with the injection of foreign substances. JAMA 82: 1091–8

Lang D, Alpern M, Visintainer P, Smith S (1993) Elevated risk of anaphylactoid reaction from radiographic contrast media is associated with both beta blocker exposure and cardiovascular disorders. Arch Intern Med 153: 2033–40

Lang D, Alpern M, Visintainer P, Smith S (1995) Gender risk for anaphylactoid reaction to radiographic contrast media. J Allergy Clin Immunol 95: 813–17

Lasser E, Lyon S, Berry C (1997) Reports on contrast media reactions: analysis of data from reports to the US Food and Drug Administration. Radiology 203: 605–10

Laxenaire M, Mertes P (2001) Anaphylaxis during anaesthesia. Results of a two year survey in France. Br J Anaesth 87: 549–58

Leech S (2002) Applied physiology: understanding allergy. Current Paediatrics 12: 376–81

Leynadier F, Pecquet C, Dry J (1988) Anaphylaxis to latex during surgery. Anaesthesia 44: 547–50

Lieberman P, Siegle R (1999) Reactions to radio-contrast material. Anaphylactoid events in radiology. Clin Rev Allergy Immunol 17: 469–96

Littenberg B, Gluck E (1986) A controlled trial of methylprednisolone in the emergency treatment of acute asthma. N Engl J Med 314: 150–7

Maddox T (2002) Adverse reactions to contrast media: recognition, prevention and treatment. Am Fam Phys 66: 1229–34

Maulitz R, Pratt D, Schocket A (1979) Exercise-induced anaphylactic reaction to shellfish. J Allergy Clin Immunol 63(6):433–4

Michael J, Guerci A, Koeler R et al. (1984) Mechanisms by Which Epinephrine Augments Cerebral and Myocardial Perfusion during Cardiopulmonary Resuscitation in Dogs, 6th edn. Mosby, London

Minhaj S, Teuber S (1998) Epinephrine is not routinely prescribed for systemic reactions caused by foods. J Allergy Clin Immunol 101: S94

Montanaro A, Bardana E Jr (2002) The mechanisms, causes and treatment of anaphylaxis. J Invest Allergol Clin Immunol 12: 2–11

Moscati R, Moore G (1990) Comparison of cimetidine and diphenhydramine in the treatment of acute urticaria. Ann Emerg Med 19: 12–15

Moulton C, Yates D (1999) Lecture Notes on Emergency Medicine. Blackwell Science, Oxford

Nakamura I, Hori S, Funabiki T et al. (2002) Cardiopulmonary arrest induced by anaphylactoid reaction with contrast media. Resuscitation 53: 223–6

Nakayama T, Aizawa C, Kuno-Sakai H (1999) A clinical analysis of gelatin allergy and determination of its causal relationship to the previous administration of gelatin-containing acellular pertussis vaccine combined with diphtheria and tetanus toxoids. J Allergy Clin Immunol 103: 321–5

NMC (2002) Guidelines for Records and Record Keeping. NMC, London

Noon L (1911) Prophylactic inoculation against hay fever. Lancet 1: 1572

Novembre E, Cianferoni A, Bernardini R et al. (1998) Anaphylaxis in children: clinical and allergologic features. Pediatrics 101: 8

Parham P (2000) The Immune System. Garland Publishing, London

Patel L, Radivan FS, David TJ (1994) Management of anaphylactic reactions to food. Arch Dis Child 71: 370–5

Patja A, Makinen-Kiljunen S, Davidkin I et al. (2001) Allergic reactions to measles–mumps–rubella vaccination. Pediatrics 107: 27

Peebles R, Adkinson N (2000) Hypersensitivity to antibiotics. In: Schlossberg D (ed) Current Therapy of Infectious Disease. Mosby, St Louis

Perkins D, Keith P (2002) Food and exercise induced anaphylaxis: importance of history in diagnosis. Ann Allergy, Asthma Immunol 89: 15–23

Pierce L (1995) Guide to Mechanical Ventilation and Intensive Respiratory Care. WB Saunders, London

Place B (1998) Pulse oximetry in adults. Nurs Times 94: 48–9

Ponvert C, Le Clainche L, de Blic J et al. (1999) Allergy to beta-lactam antibiotics in children. Pediatrics 104: 4

Pool V, Braun M, Kelso J et al. (2002) Prevalence of anti-gelatin IgE antibodies in people with anaphylaxis after measles–mumps–rubella vaccine in the United States. Pediatrics 110: 71

Portier P, Richet C (1902) De l'action anaphylactique de certains venins. C R Soc Biol (Paris) 54: 170–2

Project Team of the Resuscitation Council (UK) (1999) The emergency medical treatment of anaphylactic reactions. J Accident Emerg Med 16: 243–7

Project Team of the Resuscitation Council (UK) (2001) Update on the emergency medical treatment of anaphylactic reactions for first medical responders and for community nurses. Resuscitation 48: 241–3

Project Team of the Resuscitation Council (UK) (2002) Emergency medical treatment of anaphylactic reactions for first medical responders and for community nurses. Resuscitation Council (UK), London; accessed from www.resus.org.uk (May 2003)

Pumphrey R (2000) Lessons for management of anaphylaxis from a study of fatal reactions. Clin Exp Allergy 30: 1144–50

Pumphrey R (2003) Fatal posture in anaphylactic shock. J Allergy Clin Immunol 112: 451–2

Pumphrey R (2004) Fatal Anaphylaxis in the UK, 1992–2001. Novatis Foundation Symposium 257: 116–32

Pumphrey R, Nicholls J (2000) Epinephrine-resistant food anaphylaxis. Lancet 355: 1099.

Pumphrey R, Roberts I (2000) Postmortem findings after fatal anaphylactic reactions. J Clin Path 53: 273–6

Pumphrey R, Stanworth S (1996) The clinical spectrum of anaphylaxis in northwest England. Clin Exp Allergy 26: 1364–70

Rainbow J, Browne G (2002) Fatal asthma or anaphylaxis? Emerg Med J 19: 415–17

Raiten D, Talbot J, Fisher K (1995) Analysis of adverse reaction to monosodium glutamate. J Nutr 125: 2892S–906S

Rees J, Price JF (1999) ABC of Asthma. BMJ Books, London

Reider N, Kretz B, Menardi G et al. (2002) Outcome of a latex avoidance program in a high-risk population for latex allergy – a five-year follow-up study. Clin Exp Allergy 32: 708–13

Reisman R (1992) Stinging insect allergy. Med Clin North Am 76: 883–94

Reisman R, Livingston A (1989) Late onset allergic reactions, including serum sickness after insect stings. J Allergy Clin Immunol 84: 331

Resuscitation Council (UK) (2000a) Advanced Life Support Manual, 4th edn. Resuscitation Council (UK), London

Resuscitation Council (UK) (2000b) Resuscitation Guidelines 2000. Resuscitation Council (UK), London

Ring J, Darsow U (2002) Idiopathic anaphylaxis. Current Allergy & Asthma Reports 2(1): 40–5

Roberts J, Wuerz R (1991) Clinical characteristics of angiotensin converting enzyme inhibitor-induced angioedema. Ann Emerg Med 20: 555–8

Roitt I (1997) Essential Immunology, 9th edn. Blackwell Science, Oxford

Rose M, Fisher M (2001) Rocuronium: high risk for anaphylaxis? Br J Anaesth 86: 678–82

Royal College of Radiologists (1991) Guidelines for Use of Low Osmolar Contrast Media. Royal College of Radiologists, London

Royal College of Radiologists (1996) Advice on the Management of Reactions to Intravenous Contrast Media. Royal College of Radiologists, London

Runge J, Martinez J, Caravati E et al. (1992) Histamine antagonists in the treatment of allergic reactions. Ann Emerg Med 21: 237–42

Rusznak C, Davies R (2000) Diagnosing allergy. In: Durham S (ed) ABC of Allergies. BMJ Books, London

Rusznak C, Peebles R (2002) Anaphylaxis and anaphylactoid reactions. Postgrad Med 111

Saff R, Nahhas A, Fink J (1993) Myocardial infarction induced by coronary vasospasm after self-administration of epinephrine. Ann Allergy 70: 396–8

Sakaguchi M, Inouye I (2001) Anaphylaxis to gelatin-containing rectal suppositories. J Allergy Clin Immunol 108: 1033–4

Sakaguchi M, Nakayama T, Inouye S (1996) Food allergy to gelatin in children with systemic immediate-type reactions, including anaphylaxis, to vaccines. J Allergy Clin Immunol 98: 1058–61

Sampson H (1992) Fatal and near-fatal anaphylactic reactions to food in children and adolescents. N Engl J Med 327: 380–4

Sampson H (1999) Food allergy. Part 1: immunopathogenesis and clinical disorders. J Allergy Clin Immunol 103: 717–28

Schierhout G, Roberts I (1998) Fluid resuscitation with colloid or crystalloid solutions in critically ill patients: a systematic review of randomised trials. Br Med J 316: 961–4

Schwartz L, Bradford T, Rouse C et al. (1994) Development of a new, more sensitive immunoassay for human tryptase: use in systemic anaphylaxis. J Clin Immunol 14: 190–204

Schwartz H, Yunginger J, Schwartz L (1995a) Is unrecognised anaphylaxis a cause of sudden unexpected death? Clin Exp Allergy 25: 966–70

Schwartz L, Sakai K, Bradford T et al. (1995b) The alpha form of human tryptase is the predominant type present in blood at baseline in normal subjects and is elevated in those with systemic mastocytosis. J Clin Invest 96: 2702–10

Sen I, Mitra S, Gombar K (2001) Fatal anaphylactic reaction to oral diclofenac sodium [letter]. Can J Anaesth 48: 421

Settipane G, Chafee F, Klein D et al. (1980) Anaphylactic reactions to hymenoptera stings in asthmatic patients. Clin Allergy 10: 659–65

Shadick N, Liang M, Partridge A et al. (1999) The natural history of exercise-induced anaphylaxis: survey results from a 10 year follow-up study. J Allergy Clin Immunol 104: 123–7

Shehadi W (1985) Death following intravenous administration of contrast media. Act Radiol Diagn 26: 457–61

Sheikh A, Alves B (2000) Hospital admissions for acute anaphylaxis: time trend study. Br Med J 320: 1441

Sheikh A, Alves B (2001) Age, sex, geographical and socio-economic variations in admission for anaphylaxis: analysis of four years of English hospital data. Clin Exp Allergy 31: 1571–6

Sherwood L (2001) Human Physiology from Cells to Systems, 4th edn. Brooks/Cole, UK

Shimamoto S, Bock S (2003) Update on the clinical features of food-induced anaphylaxis. Curr Opin Allergy Clin Immunol 2: 211–16

Shingai Y, Nakagawa K, Kato T et al. (2002) Severe allergy in a pregnant woman after vaginal examination with a latex glove. Gynecol Obstet Invest 54: 183–4

Sicherer S (2003) Advances in anaphylaxis and hypersensitivity reactions to foods, drugs and insect venom. J Allergy Clin Immunol 111(3 Suppl): S829–34

Sicherer S, Forman J, Noone S (2000) Use assessment of self-administered epinephrine among food-allergic children and pediatricians. Pediatrics 105: 359–62

Simon R, Brenner B (1994) Emergency Procedures and Techniques in Airway Procedures. Williams & Wilkins, London

Simons F, Robert J, Gu X, Simons K (1998) Epinephrine absorption in children with a history of anaphylaxis. J Allergy Clin Immunol 101: 33–7

Simons F, Gu X, Johnston L, Simons K (2000) Can epinephrine inhalations be substituted for epinephrine injection in children at risk for severe anaphylaxis? Pediatrics 106: 1040–4

Simons F, Gu X, Simons K (2001) Epinephrine absorption in adults: intramuscular versus subcutaneous injection. J Allergy Clin Immunol 108: 871–3

Simons F, Peterson S, Black C (2002b) Epinephrine dispensing patterns for an out-of-hospital population: a novel approach to studying the epidemiology of anaphylaxis. J Allergy Clin Immunol 110: 647–51

Simons F, Gu X, Silver N, Simons K (2002a) EpiPen Jr versus EpiPen in young children weighing 15–30 kg at risk for anaphylaxis. J Allergy Clin Immunol 109: 171–5

Smoley B (2002) Oropharyngeal hymenoptera stings: a special concern for airway obstruction. Military Med 167: 161–3

Snyder H, Weiss E (1989) Hysterical stridor: a benign cause of upper airway obstruction. Ann Emerg Med 18: 991

Staines N, Brostoff J, James K (1993) Introducing Immunology. Mosby, London

Statement from the Resuscitation Council (UK) and the Joint Royal Colleges Ambulance Service Liaison Committee (1997) The use of adrenaline for anaphylactic shock (for ambulance paramedics). Ambulance UK 12: 16

Steensma D (2003) The kiss of death: a severe allergic reaction to shellfish induced by a goodnight kiss. Mayo Clin Proc 78: 221–2

Stewart A, Ewan P (1996) The incidence, aetiology and management of anaphylaxis presenting to an accident and emergency department. QJ Med 89: 859

Sussman G, Tarlo S, Dolovich J (1992) The spectrum of IgE-mediated responses to latex. JAMA 265: 2844–7

Sutton B, Gould H (1993) The human IgE network. Nature 366: 421–8

Tan B, Sher M, Good A, Bahna S (2001) Severe food allergies by skin contact. Ann Allergy, Asthma Immunol 86: 583–6

Tariq S, Stevens M, Matthews S et al. (1996) Cohort study of peanut and tree nut sensitisation by age of 4 years. Br Med J 313: 514–17

Technology Subcommittee of the Working Group on Critical Care (1992) Non-invasive blood gas monitoring: a review for use in the adult critical care unit. Can Med Assoc J 146: 703–12

Tejedor A, Sastre D, Sanchez-Hernandez J, Perez F (2002) Idiopathic anaphylaxis: a descriptive study of 81 patients in Spain. Ann Allergy, Asthma Immunol 88: 313–18

Tierney L, McPhee S, Papadakis M (2002) Current Medical Diagnosis & Treatment, 41st edn. Lange Medical Books/McGraw-Hill, London

Toogood J (1988) Risk of anaphylaxis in patients receiving beta-blocker drugs. J Allergy Clin Immunol 81: 1–5

Unsworth D (2001) Adrenaline syringes are vastly over-prescribed. Arch Dis Child 84: 410–11

Valentine M, Schuberth K, Kagey-Sobotka A et al. (1990) The value of immunotherapy with venom in children with allergy to insect stings. N Engl J Med 323: 1601–3

van Puijenbroek E, Egberts A, Meyboom R, Leufkens H (2002) Different risks for NSAID-induced anaphylaxis. Ann Pharmacother 36: 24–9

Vanin E, Zanconato S, Baraldi E, Marcazzo L (2002) Anaphylactic reaction after skin-prick testing in an 8-year old boy. Pediatr Allergy Immunol 13: 227–8

Vervloet D, Durham S (2000) Adverse reactions to drugs. In: Durham S (ed) ABC of Allergies. BMJ Books, London

Vickers D, Maynard L, Ewan P (1997) Management of children with potential anaphylactic reactions in the community: a training package and proposal for good practice. Clin Exp Allergy 27: 898–903

Visscher P, Vetter R, Camazine S (1996) Removing bee stings. Lancet 348: 301–2

Volcheck G (2002) Hymenoptera (apid and vespid) allergy; update in diagnosis and management. Curr Allergy Asthma Rep 2: 46–50

Wakelin S (2002) Contact anaphylaxis from natural rubber latex used as an adhesive for hair extensions [Letter]. Br J Dermatol 146: 340–1

Waugh A, Grant A (2001) Ross and Wilson's Anatomy and Physiology in Health and Illness, 9th edn. Churchill Livingstone, Edinburgh

Waytes A, Rosen F, Frank M (1996) Treatment of hereditary angioedema with vapor-heated C-1 inhibitor concentrate. N Engl J Med 334: 1630–4

Weiler J (1999) Anaphylaxis in the general population. A frequent and occasionally fatal disorder that is under recognised. J Allergy Clin Immunol 104: 271

Wensing M, Knulst A, Piersma S et al. (2003) Patients with anaphylaxis to pea can have peanut allergy caused by cross-reactive IgE to vicilin. J Allergy Clin Immunol 111: 420–4

Williams J (2002) The management of food allergy in children. Current Paediatrics 12: 365–9

Wilson R (2000) Upward trend in acute anaphylaxis continued in 1998–9. Br Med J 321: 1021

Wong D, Hockenberry-Eaton M, Wilson D et al. (1999) Nursing Care of Infants and Children, 6th edn. Mosby, London

Woods J, Lambert S, Platts-Mills T et al. (1997) Natural rubber latex allergy: spectrum, diagnostic approach and therapy. J Emerg Med 15: 71–85

Wynn K (1998) Going latex safe. Arch Intern Med 6: 44–9

Wynn S, Frazier C, Munozfurlong A et al. (1993) Anaphylaxis at school: etiological factors, prevalence and treatment. Pediatrics 91: 516

Yarbrough J, Moffitt J, Brown D et al. (1989) Cimetidine in the treatment of refractory anaphylaxis. Ann Allergy 63: 235–8

Yocum M, Butterfield J et al. (1999) Epidemiology of anaphylaxis in Olmsted County: a population-based study. J Allergy Clin Immunol 104: 452

Yunginger J (1998) Insect allergy. In: Middleton E Jr et al. (eds) Allergy: Principles and Practice. Mosby, St Louis

Yunginger J (1999) Latex allergy in the workplace: an overview of where we are. Ann Allergy Asthma Immunol 83: 630–3

Yunginger J, Sweeney K, Sturner W et al. (1988) Fatal food-induced anaphylaxis. JAMA 260: 1450–2

Yunginger J, Nelson D, Squilace D et al. (1991) Laboratory investigation of deaths due to anaphylaxis. J Forensic Sci 36: 857–65

Zacharisen M, Elms N, Kurup V (2002) Severe tomato allergy. Allergy Asthma Proc 23: 149–52

Zideman D, Spearpoint K (1999) Resuscitation of infants and children. In: Colquhoun M et al. (eds) ABC of Resuscitation, 4th edn. BMJ Books, London

Zull D (1999) Anaphylaxis. In: Schwartz G (ed) Principles and Practice of Emergency Medicine, 4th edn. Wilkins & Wilkins, London

Index